LEELANAU BY KAYAK

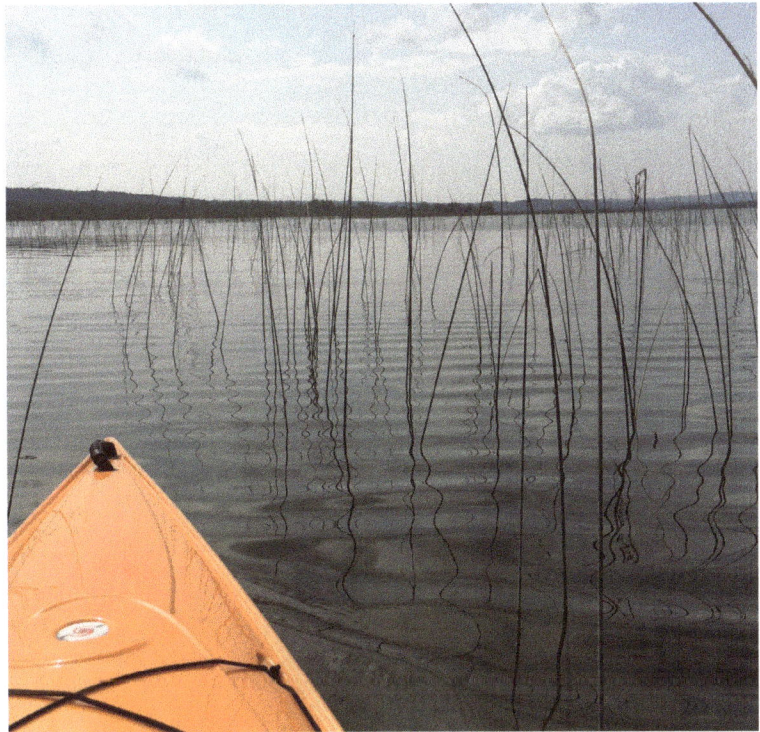

For my grandchildren, Caden Jon and Camryn Jolene Bogard. May there always be beautiful and pristine waters in the Leelanau region for both you and your friends to enjoy.

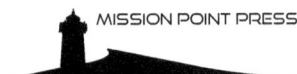

MISSION POINT PRESS

Published by Mission Point Press
2554 Chandler Rd.
Traverse City, MI 49696
(231) 421-9513
www.MissionPointPress.com

ISBN: 978-1-943995-62-2
Library of Congress Control Number:
2018938955

Printed in the United States of America

I would like to give a heartfelt thanks to everyone who helped me with this book. A special thank you goes out to Dick and Pat Hatfield for their generous support, and for Pat's expert suggestions on my text. Also, a big thank you to Doug Weaver and everyone at Mission Point Press who helped guide me in this project, especially to Heather Shaw who did an amazing job in designing, editing and producing this book and making it as good as I think it could be. This has certainly been a very interesting journey.

All the photos in the book were taken by the author. The three exceptions are: the photo on page 11 that was taken by a friendly passerby on the Leland beach; the photo on page 36 by David Clinton; and the photo on page 143 by Kacie Constant Bogard.

Some of the facts on the rivers and lakes of Leelanau were from Jim Stamm's book, *A Guide to the Rivers and Lakes of Grand Traverse And Leelanau Counties, Michigan*, and are used by permission.

The map opposite the Table of Contents, was used with the permission of Michigan Maps Inc, (Mark Stone), P.O. Box 885 Elk Rapids, Michigan, 49629.

The other maps were used with permission of Mapping Unlimited, (Butch and Linda Hoogerhyde), 6235 Crystal Springs Road, Bellaire, Michigan, 49615.

Frontcover photo taken at the Leland Clay Cliffs (June 10, 2018)

Backcover photo taken on Cedar Lake (June 12, 2018)

LEELANAU BY KAYAK

DAY TRIPS, PICS, TIPS, AND STORIES OF A BEAUTIFUL PENINSULA

JON R. CONSTANT
with LARRY BURNS

EXPANDED SECOND EDITION

MISSION POINT PRESS

Leelanau County, Michigan

General Reference Map
Depicting Land and Water in Physical Relief

LAND RELIEF (in Meters)

- 380-400 m.
- 360-380 m.
- 340-360 m.
- 320-340 m.
- 300-320 m.
- 280-300 m.
- 260-280 m.
- 240-260 m.
- 220-240 m.
- 200-220 m.
- 180-200 m.
- 177-180 m.

INLAND LAKE DEPTH

- 0-5 ft.
- 5-10 ft.
- 10-20 ft.
- 20-40 ft.
- 40-60 ft.
- 60-80 ft.
- 80-100 ft.
- 100-120 ft.
- 120-135 ft.

GREAT LAKES DEPTH (in Feet)

- 0-5 ft.
- 5-15 ft.
- 15-30 ft.
- 30-60 ft.
- 60-120 ft.
- 120-300 ft.
- Over 300 ft.

Legend

- Local Park
- National/State Park
- Public Campground
- Nature Preserve
- Picnic Area/Rest Stop
- Scenic Overlook
- Trailhead-Snowmobile
- Trailhead-ORV
- Trailhead-Hike
- Trailhead-X-Country (Ski)
- Trailhead-Bike
- Swimming Area
- Fishing Access
- Canoe Access
- Boat Ramp
- Marina/Harbor
- Lighthouse
- Airstrip
- Airport
- Ferry Dock
- Hospital
- Tourist Info
- Gov't. Office
- County Seat
- Ranger/Police
- Museum/Library
- College/School
- Church
- Cemetery
- Mine/Quarry
- Playing Field/Stadium
- Golf Course
- Point of Interest
- Federal Interstate
- Federal Highway
- State Highway
- County Primary
- Principal Local Road
- Other Roads/Trails
- Railroad
- Snowmobile Trail
- ORV Trail
- Non-Motorized Trail
- Multi-Purpose Trail
- Interchange
- Settlement/Village
- County Boundary
- Township Boundary
- Latitude/Longitude Line

Leelanau County Statistics

Area	348 sq. mi.
Population (2000)	21,119
Pop. Increase (1990-2000)	27.9%
Median Household Income (03)	$50,150
Median Home Value (2000)	$165,400

Source: U.S. Census Bureau

North Manitou Island
South Manitou Island
Lake Michigan
Grand Traverse Bay

NORTHPORT
LELAND
PESHAWBESTOWN
SUTTONS BAY
LAKE LEELANAU
GLEN ARBOR
GLEN HAVEN
BURDICKVILLE
MAPLE CITY
CEDAR
EMPIRE
GREILICKVILLE
TRAVERSE CITY
ACME

I# LEPR18 ver. 1.1
by Mark Stone

CONTENTS

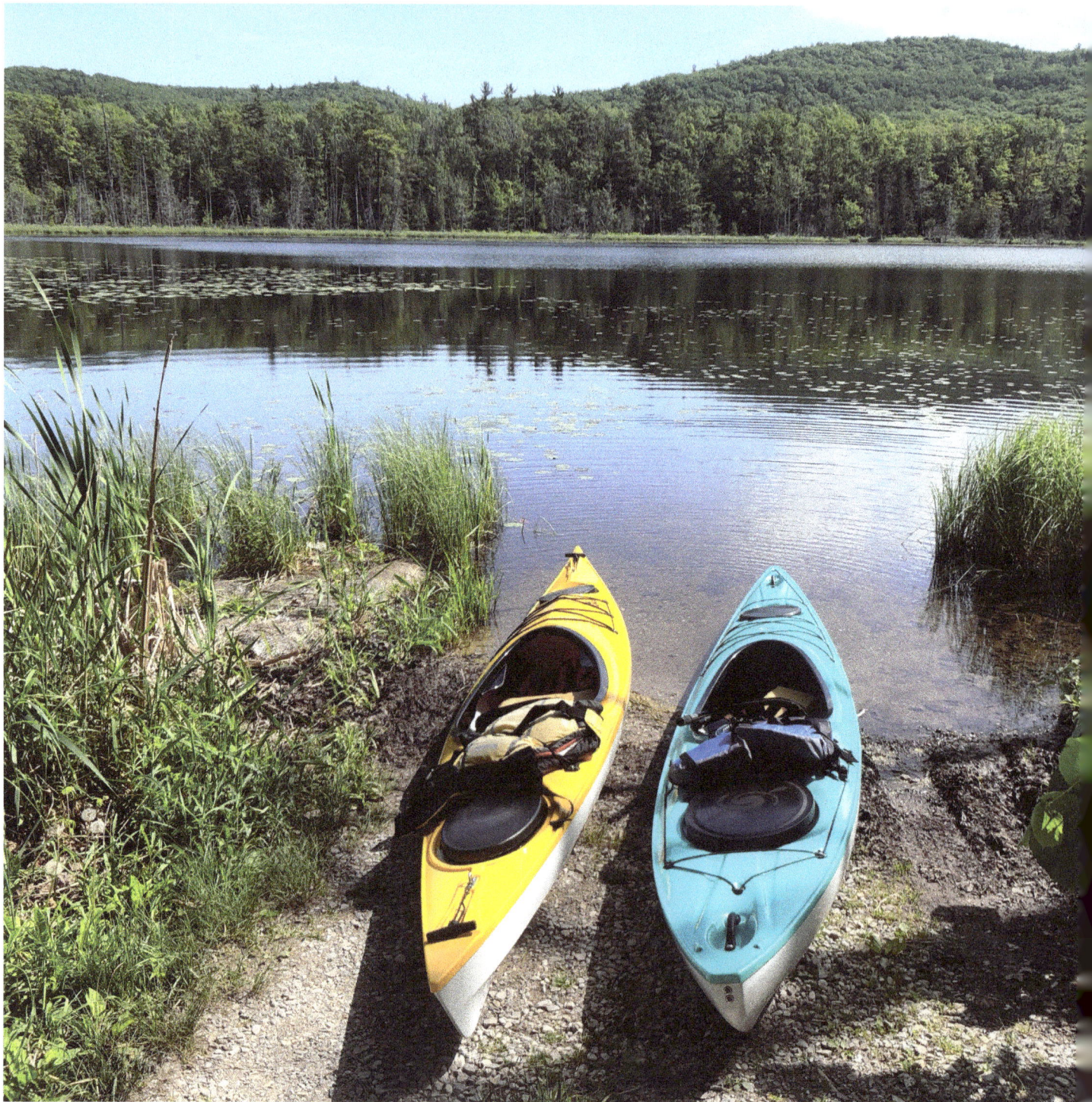

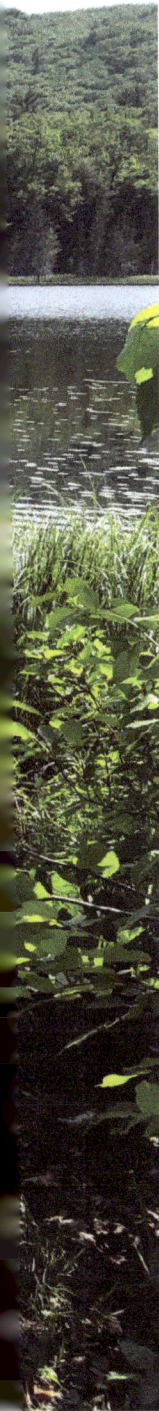

THOUGHTS ON THE SECOND EDITION

Writing the book *Leelanau By Kayak* has been a wonderful experience and a lot of fun for me and I think that the book came out much better than I could ever have imagined. So then, why do a second edition? Here are a few of the reasons:

- First, there were a few small lakes in Leelanau that we hadn't paddled and therefore were not included in the first book. Well, in 2018 we got to paddle Davis Lake, Armstrong Lake, Kehl Lake, and we tried mightily to get on Woolsey Lake. All of them are now included in this edition of the book.

- Secondly, we had an amazing kayaking season in 2018! Larry and I were able to return to many of our favorite locations, including Leelanau's Big Four: the Empire Bluffs, The Big Bear at the Sleeping Bear Dunes, Pyramid Point and the Leland Clay Cliffs. Some of those experiences are in this edition.

- Thirdly, this edition includes over 20 new photos from 2018 and earlier seasons. I would like to thank Shelly Miller Engel of Spring Lake, Michigan, and Dick Hatfield of Carrboro, North Carolina, who helped me in selecting the new photos. They are two of my "Class of 1968" Grand Haven High School classmates. Go Bucs!

- Also, the section "Practical Matters" was moved from the beginning of the book to just before "Last Words" where I believe it is a better fit.

- And lastly, the season of kayaking after the 1st edition was published has given us another paddling season of experience that we can share. One important example involves the issue of kayaking safety. Larry and I both had separate minor "incidents" in 2018— each one that could have ended up much worse. My accident occurred on West Bay boat launch when I was hurried and pulled up my kayak too quickly. I slipped on some very slimy rocks and fell backward, my lower back hitting a stump. I was OK, but I wasn't quite so sure for a minute or two. Larry's kayaking incident involved his kayak getting caught up in a Crystal River current. Both cases were reminders for us, and for you, to be safe. If you plan on enjoying the beauty of Leelanau's waters from your kayak…do so carefully.

For all these reasons, I hope you enjoy the second edition of *Leelanau By Kayak*.

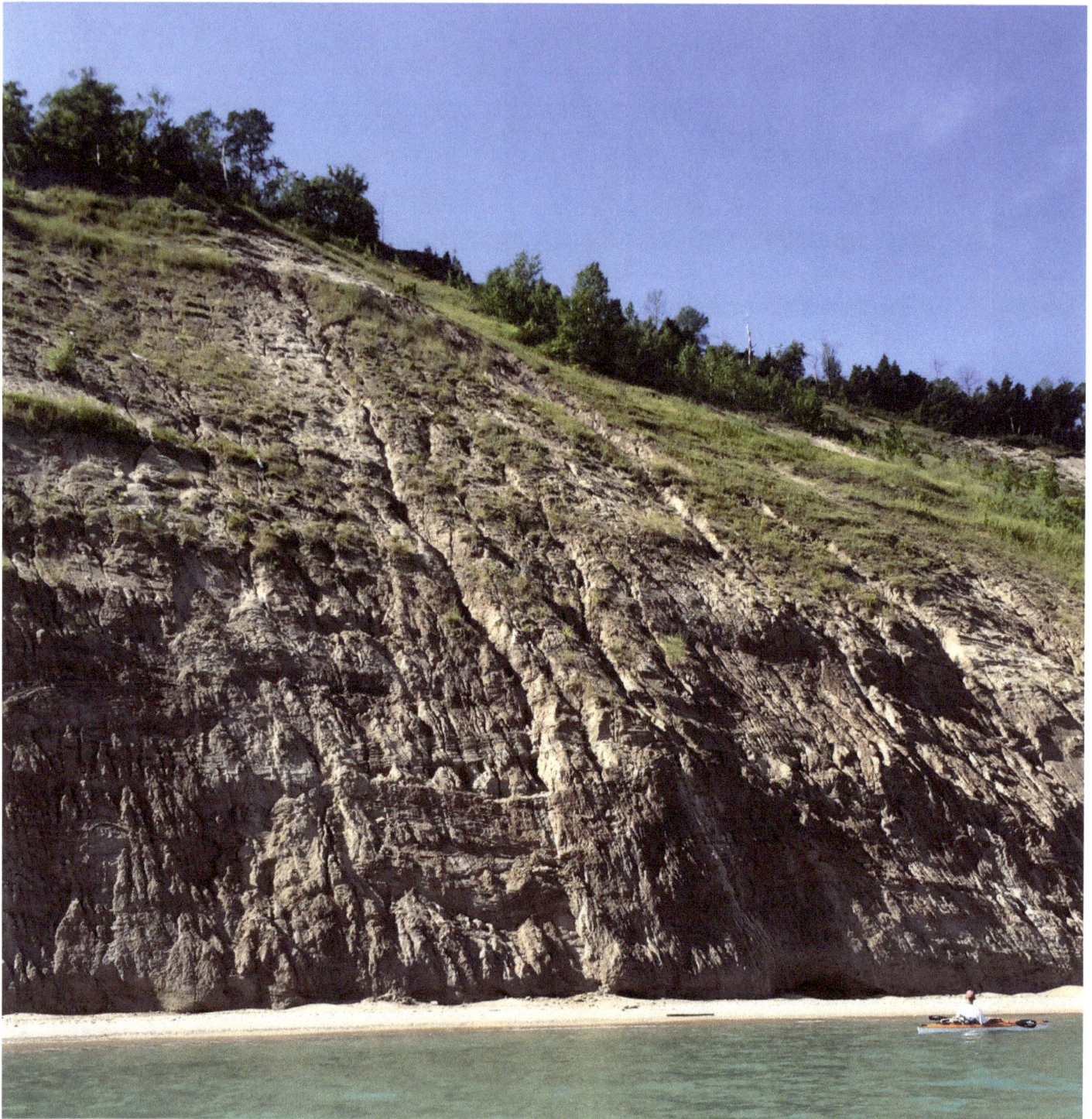

INTRODUCTION

This is a book about kayaking. This is also a book about the Leelanau Peninsula. There are many books about kayaking, and there are many books about the beauty of Leelanau, but this book is probably the only one that is about both kayaking and the wonders of Leelanau.

My connection to the water goes back a long way. I grew up in Grand Haven, Michigan, which is located on Lake Michigan, at the mouth of the Grand River. The house I grew up in was on Robbins Road, and less than a mile from the Big Lake —well within the sound of its waves, when the lake was rough, or the foghorn on the Grand Haven pier. As a teenager, I bought an old, 15-foot wooden boat with a red 15-horse Johnson outboard motor and docked it for a few years on the Grand River. I had a great time exploring the Grand River channels, the river's bayous, Spring Lake and, a few times, venturing out into Lake Michigan. I guess that I was a regular Huck Finn or Tom Sawyer. I also have many memories of our family going to "The Oval," which is now called the Grand Haven State Park, for picnics, swims or just to look at the sunset. I still make an effort to drive along the roads that go past the river, the park and Lake Michigan every time I visit my hometown. Growing up, I always said that if I could, I would love to live on a lake and explore the water of Michigan. I have been so lucky to be able to live that dream.

My dad was a teacher at Grand Haven High School, and I took his Michigan History class. I distinctly remember sitting in that class in the 1960s, listening to him talk about the early Native Americans and the French fur traders. I thought a lot about what it must have been like in those days. He said that the name for the French explorers was *Les Coureur des Bois* (the runners of the woods), and that they were a tough and hardy group. They paddled the rivers, lakes and bays of what is now Michigan in pursuit of fur and fortune. I would sit in his class and dream about how and where they had paddled their canoes and dug-out boats. My dad would also talk of the early settlers who came west into Michigan on wooden schooners. Now, when I am paddling the waters around Leelanau, I often think that the same water and the scenery I am seeing is like the views that these earlier people saw. I eventually followed in my dad's footsteps and also became a high school history teacher. All this may help explain why I have included a little bit of the history of some of the places we paddled by in Leelanau.

Before we begin, let me say that it took a few very unlikely things coming together for this book to come together.

First, I do not make the claim that I am an expert kayaker. My first kayaking experience was probably like many of yours — I just got in a kayak on a nice, summer day on a quiet lake and started paddling. You have to start somewhere. Full disclosure: I have never had any lessons or training, although I do recommend doing so. What I have done is read many books and articles on kayaking by others who are expert paddlers. I was also lucky enough to have found a paddling partner like Larry Burns, who was and is a much better kayaker. Larry had more experience kayaking than me, and I have learned much about the sport from him. Therefore, although I do not claim to be a kayaking expert, I do think I have learned enough for my advice and information to be considered.

Secondly, Larry and I were able to accomplish kayaking the entire perimeter of Leelanau and its lakes and rivers in our mid to late 60s. The fact we were able to do so in our "more mature" years was actually an advantage. Because we were retired, we could more easily pick and choose the days with the best paddling conditions. An additional advantage to being retired is that we could take the next day "off" if we needed to rest some sore muscles.

The third unlikely thing about this book is that it is about kayaking just the Leelanau Peninsula. There are lots of great places to kayak in northern Michigan, and we have been to some of them. Even so, Leelanau County became our "go to location" for kayaking.

Larry and I began our kayaking day trip locations in a random fashion. Actually, paddling the entire 100 miles of the Leelanau coast, or even most of its lakes and all three of its rivers, did not begin as a goal of ours. Our initial focus on Leelanau was a practical one — traveling in the summer to sites in Leelanau means you don't have to fight the traffic that can be intense in and around Traverse City. But we were also drawn to the splendid beauty of the peninsula they call "Michigan's Little Finger." Why go anywhere else when you can paddle the stunningly magnificent waters of Leelanau? After several kayaking seasons, I was looking at my maps and made the serendipitous discovery that we were only a few day trips away from the cool achievement of paddling the entire perimeter of Leelanau and most of Leelanau's inland waters. Paddling all of Leelanau then did become our goal.

The fourth unlikely thing about this book is that I am definitely not a professional photographer. I have never taken a course on photography, nor do I even own a good camera. What I do have is an iPhone, and I have a habit of taking a lot of pictures with it. I have always taken my iPhone with me on day trips, and whenever I saw something I thought was pretty nice, I would take a picture of it. I am always surprised by how good some of the pictures look. Like most photographers will say, if you take enough pictures, some of them may turn out not so bad — and I did take a lot of pictures! I really like some of them, and I hope at least a few of them in this book look good to you, too.

The last unlikely thing about this book is that I am not a professional writer. Anyone who knows me knows that I am more of a sports guy than an artist. I have never taken a writing class outside of high school and college, but I did do some writing during my 38-year career as a high school social studies teacher at Traverse City Central High School. I hope that my experience has been the best teacher. (I do now enjoy the excuse, when I mess up around the house — like making a bigger mess than I usually do — that I can say, "Well, Mary, you married me, and you know how quirky we artists can be!")

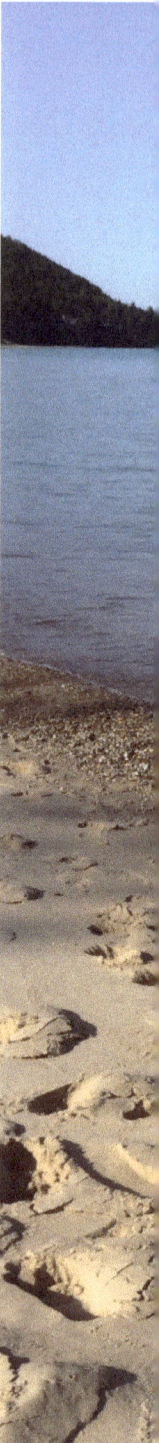

So there you have it: this is a book with photos on kayaking by an author who is not a professional kayaker, not a photographer and not a writer. If these full disclosures haven't talked you out of buying, or even looking at the book, here's the real selling point: this is a book about kayaking at some of the very best places in North America. I hope you enjoy the views as well as my story.

Jon R. Constant

_____

From its nest high atop a pine tree on the lakeside bluffs, a bald eagle swoops down, gliding over the water. You look down through the smooth, clear water and watch a bass swimming among the rocks twenty feet below. The sunlight filters through the depths, creating a sparkling, transparent scene on the sandy bottom. There is a peaceful stillness, disturbed only by the sound of the waves and the chirping of the eagle, now far overhead. The sand dunes, towering high above you along the shoreline are reflected in the ripples on the surface of the water.

You may experience much of this natural beauty and wildlife from many watercraft in many parts of the country, but for my money, paddling a kayak on the waters of Northwest Michigan is the ultimate in water sports. Sitting directly on the surface of the water while moving almost silently gives you a perspective that few boating experiences can provide. This area is a kayaker's paradise for both novice and experienced paddlers.

Do some research and find a kayak that fits your personal needs, find a friend who shares your enthusiasm and get ready for spirit lifting adventures you will not soon forget!

Larry Burns

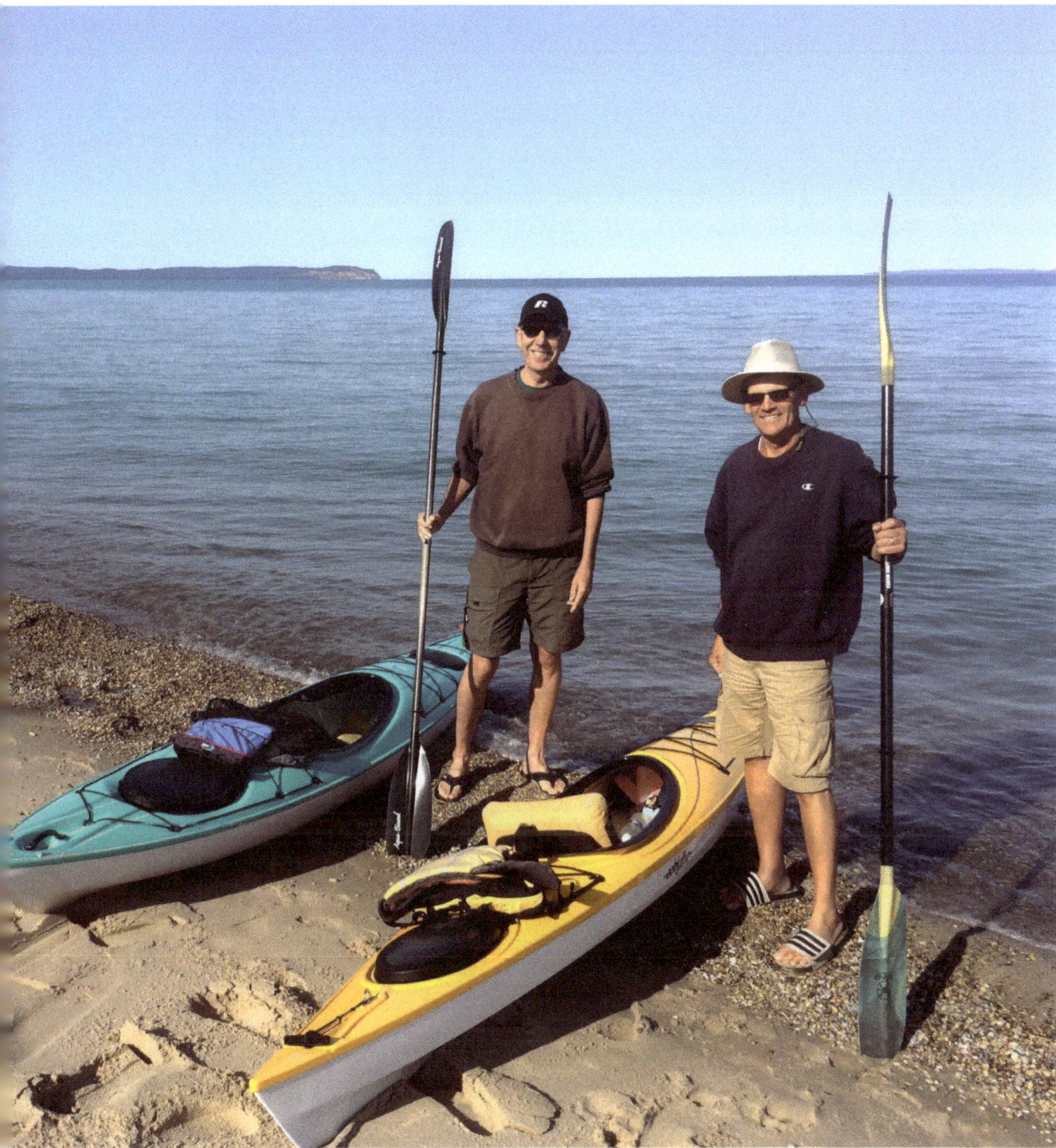

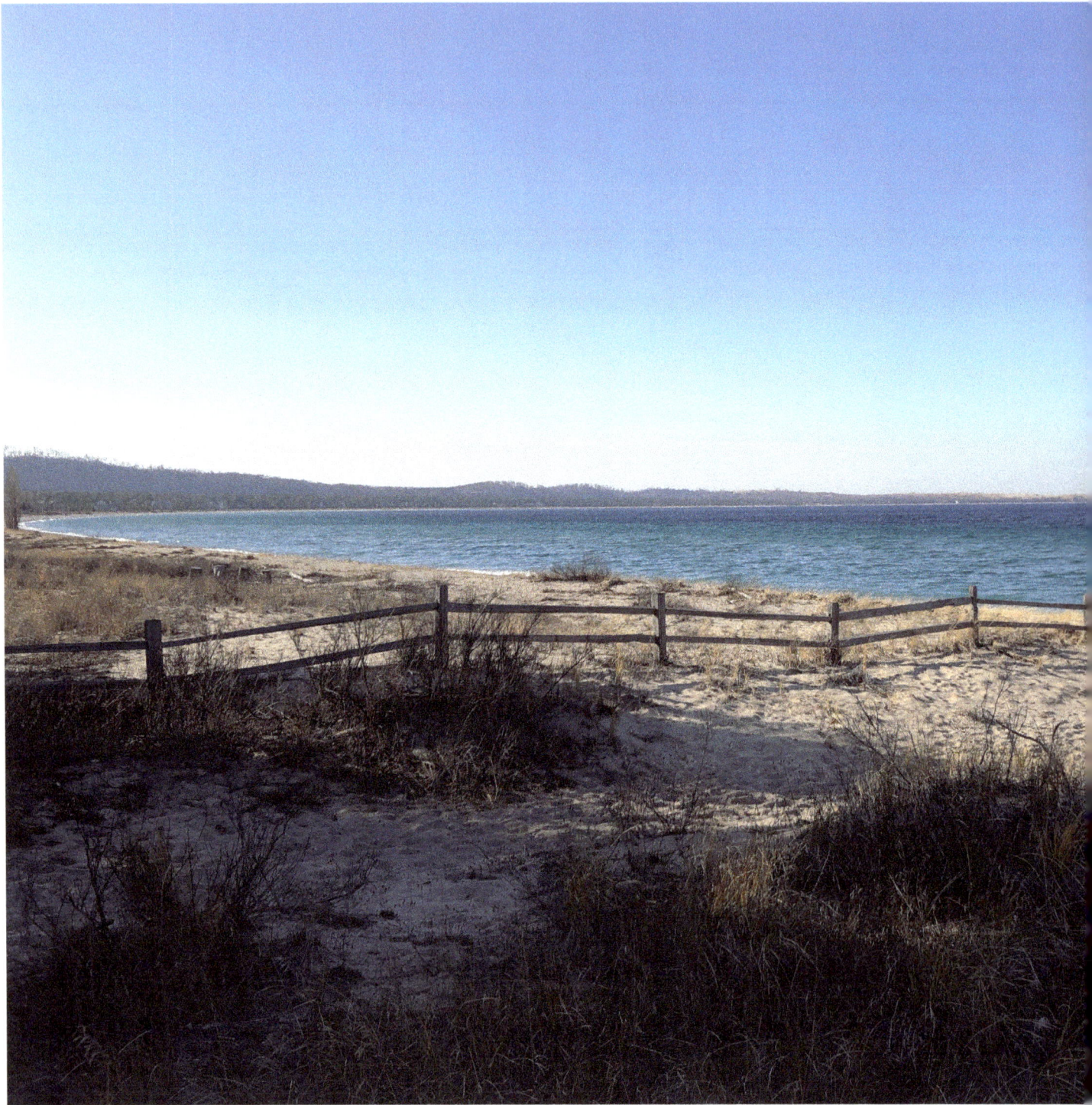

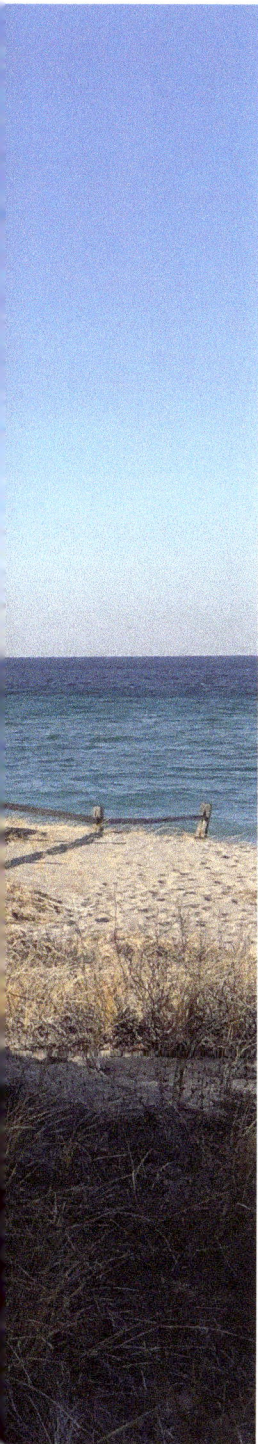

AROUND THE LEELANAU SHORELINE

The 100-mile Great Lakes shoreline of the Leelanau peninsula is beauty on a grand scale. Some of that beauty is simply the water. There may be many wonderful places to paddle in Michigan, but the clarity and the purity of the water in Leelanau is extra special. The shades of blue, green, turquoise and even purple can be stunning — especially from a kayak. Even on days when the skies are cloudy, the lake can be beautiful with its steely gray tones.

We try to go out on the Big Lake when paddling conditions are good to perfect. This means that my pictures tend to show more of the quieter side of Lake Michigan. Of course, there are other days when the lake has other moods. On those days, the beauty is best viewed from the safety of the shore.

When conditions cooperate, looking at the horizon from something as small as a kayak can really put things in perspective. Leelanau is home to massive dunes, including the bluffs south of Empire, the dunes at Sleeping Bear, Pyramid Point to the north, as well as many smaller dunes and bluffs. Also, there are incredible homes and cottages in the areas outside the National Lakeshore. In other sections there are many miles of unspoiled shoreline with sandy shores, wooded bluffs and impressive hills further inland.

We begin our journey with a trip to the Empire Bluffs, and work our way around beautiful Leelanau — one day trip at a time.

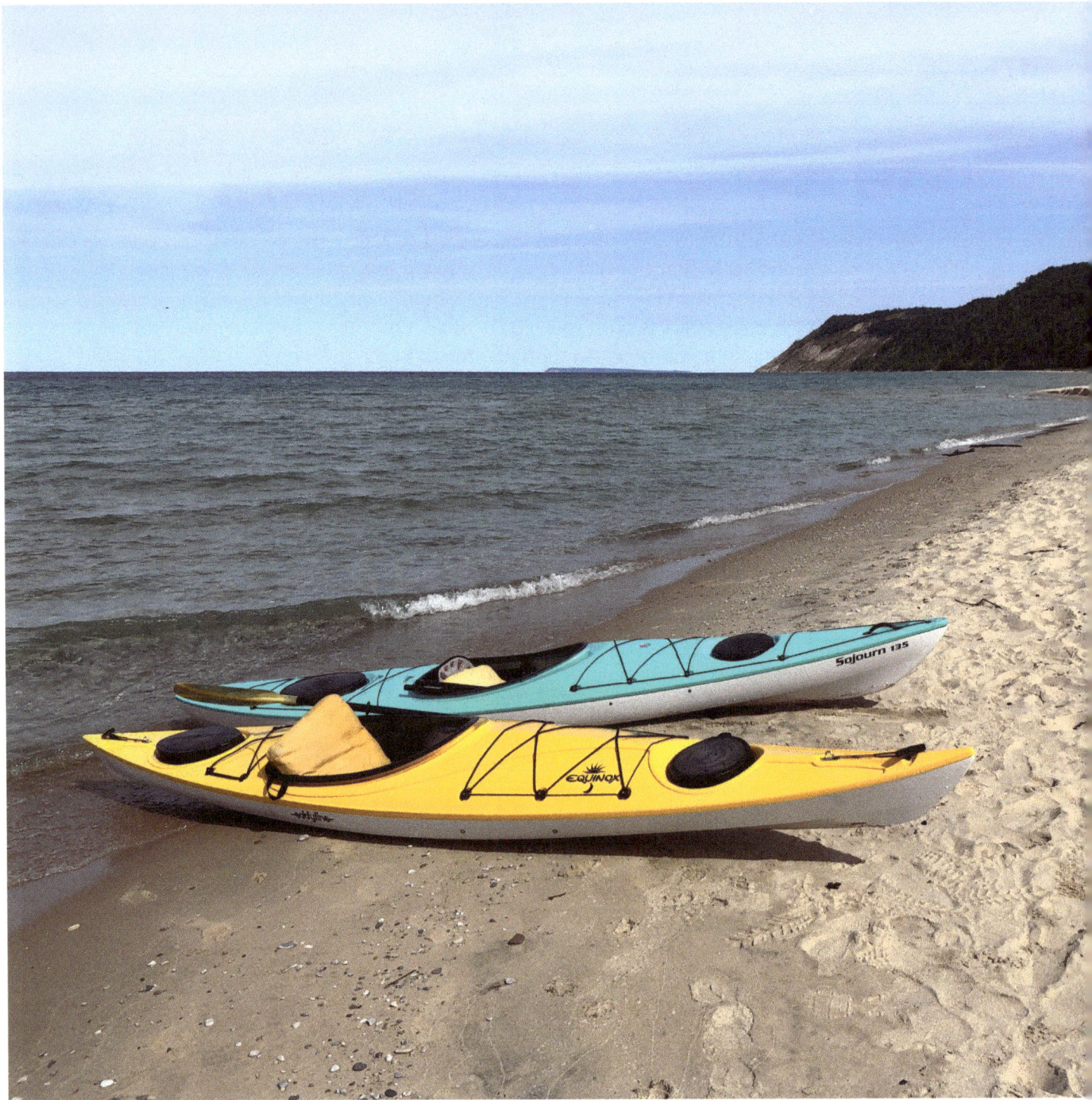

TRIP 1: EMPIRE BLUFFS

Overshadowed by the well-known Sleeping Bear Dunes and Pyramid Point to the north, the Empire Bluffs are one of the unsung gems of the entire Leelanau area. They rise 1,100 feet above sea level and over 500 feet above Lake Michigan — an impressive sight! From the water, a paddler can see the impacts of erosion and gravity, as there are many rivulets in the sand and clay, and many areas where large sections of the bluffs have slid down to the shore and lake.

This was one of our earliest ventures onto the Big Lake, and I remember my favorite part was looking north from the bluffs, with the view of the even more massive Sleeping Bear Dunes and South Manitou Island in front of us. The dunes here are unique in their own way, and the views in all directions, spectacular.

DATE OF TRIPS: August 21, 2014 and September 17, 2018

LOCATION: The southwest corner of Leelanau County, extending into Benzie County.

ACCESS: The two best access points are the Esch Road Beach and the Lake Michigan Beach Park.

- Esch Road Beach is in the Sleeping Bear Dunes National Lakeshore at the mouth of Otter Creek. It is located at the end of Esch Road, about 3 miles south of Empire on M-22. Go west on Esch Road about 1 mile to the parking area at Lake Michigan. There are bathroom facilities there. The mouth of Otter Creek moves north or south, depending on the waves on Lake Michigan, so it can be a different experience every time you go.

- Lake Michigan Beach Park is located west of the business district in the village of Empire. There are bathrooms and plenty of parking available. South Bar Lake is adjacent to the parking lot and easily accessible for a quick paddle before venturing out on the Big Lake. (For a separate paddle of its own, see page 77.) This park also features one of the newest working lighthouses on the Great Lakes!

STRATEGIES: When Larry and I paddled this section, we were using the one-vehicle system, and put it at Esch Road Beach then paddled to Empire and back. The conditions were calm and this was no problem. A better way would be to use two vehicles: putting in, then going to the dropped vehicle. This way you can go with any existing winds.

DISTANCE/TIME: The estimated distance between Esch Road Beach and Empire is about 4 miles. It took us about 2.5 hours to go round trip.

FEATURES:

» The "lost" lumber town of Aral once existed at the mouth of Otter Creek. It flourished from 1880 until the forest was depleted in the early 1900s. At one time, the two-story sawmill had 150 workers, a dock into Lake Michigan and a connecting timber tramway. There was also a schoolhouse, a post office and two boarding houses. Aral got a second life when an obscure religious sect called "The Israelite House of David" bought up the land and rebuilt the lumbering enterprise. They maintained a schooner on Lake Michigan and gave tours along the Lake Michigan coast, complete with a musical band in red uniforms. The House of David was famous for the long beards and baseball talents of their menfolk. Their local team was thought to be the best in the entire area. The House of David shut down their mill and sold off their lumber and belongings in 1911. The only thing left to see today are the pilings of the docks near the mouth of Otter Creek.

» Empire, Michigan, was founded in 1851. It was named for the schooner "Empire," which was icebound off the village in 1865. A booming lumber town in the late 1800s, Empire produced up to 20 million feet of lumber a year. Fires and depleted virgin forests ended milling operations in 1917. Today, the village of Empire has a population of 375 people and is considered an entry site for the Sleeping Bear Dunes National Lakeshore at the Philip A. Hart Visitor Center. The Robert H. Manning Memorial Lighthouse was built in 1991, and is a nice feature at the north end of the Empire Beach. Empire was also important during the Cold War as it was the site of a vital U.S. Air Force radar station.

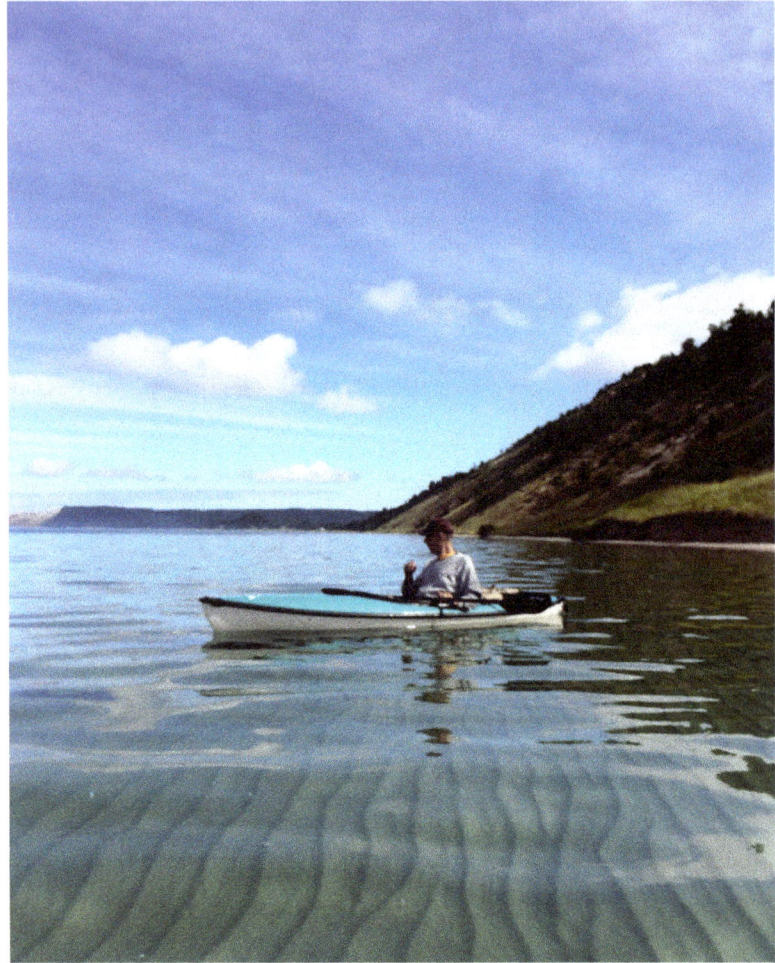

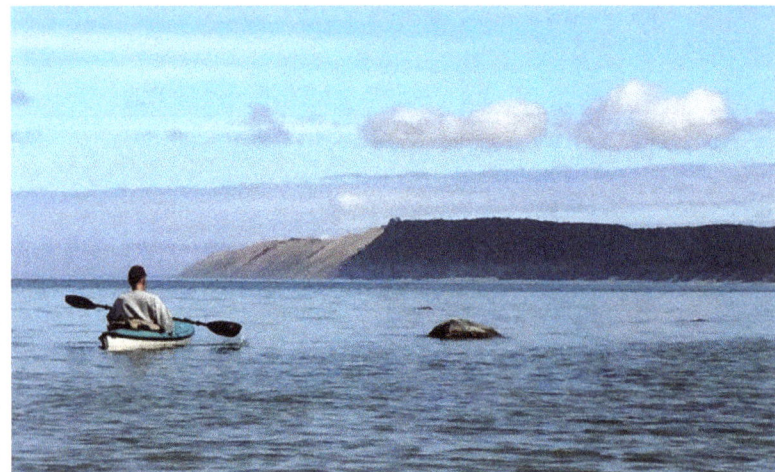

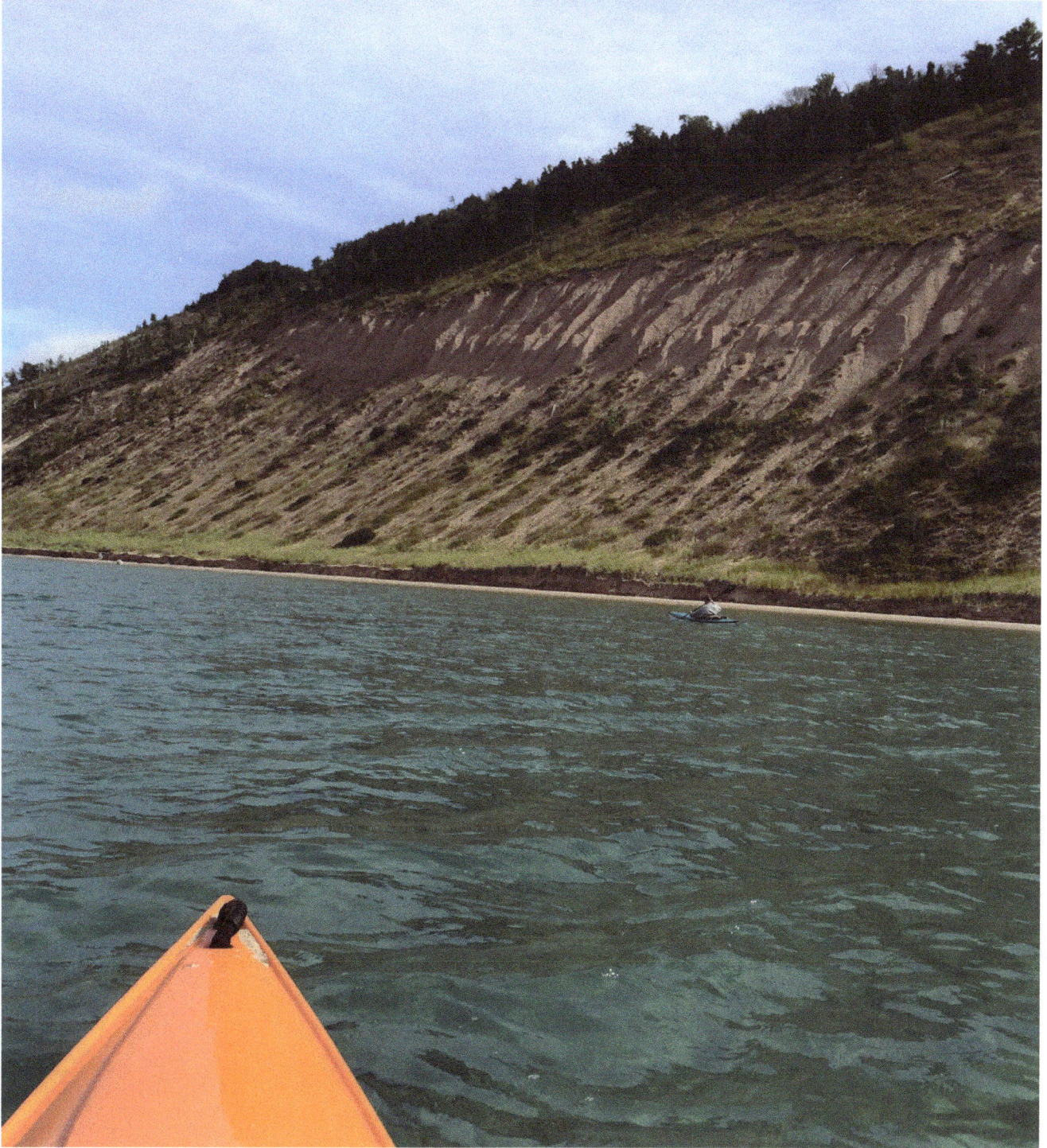

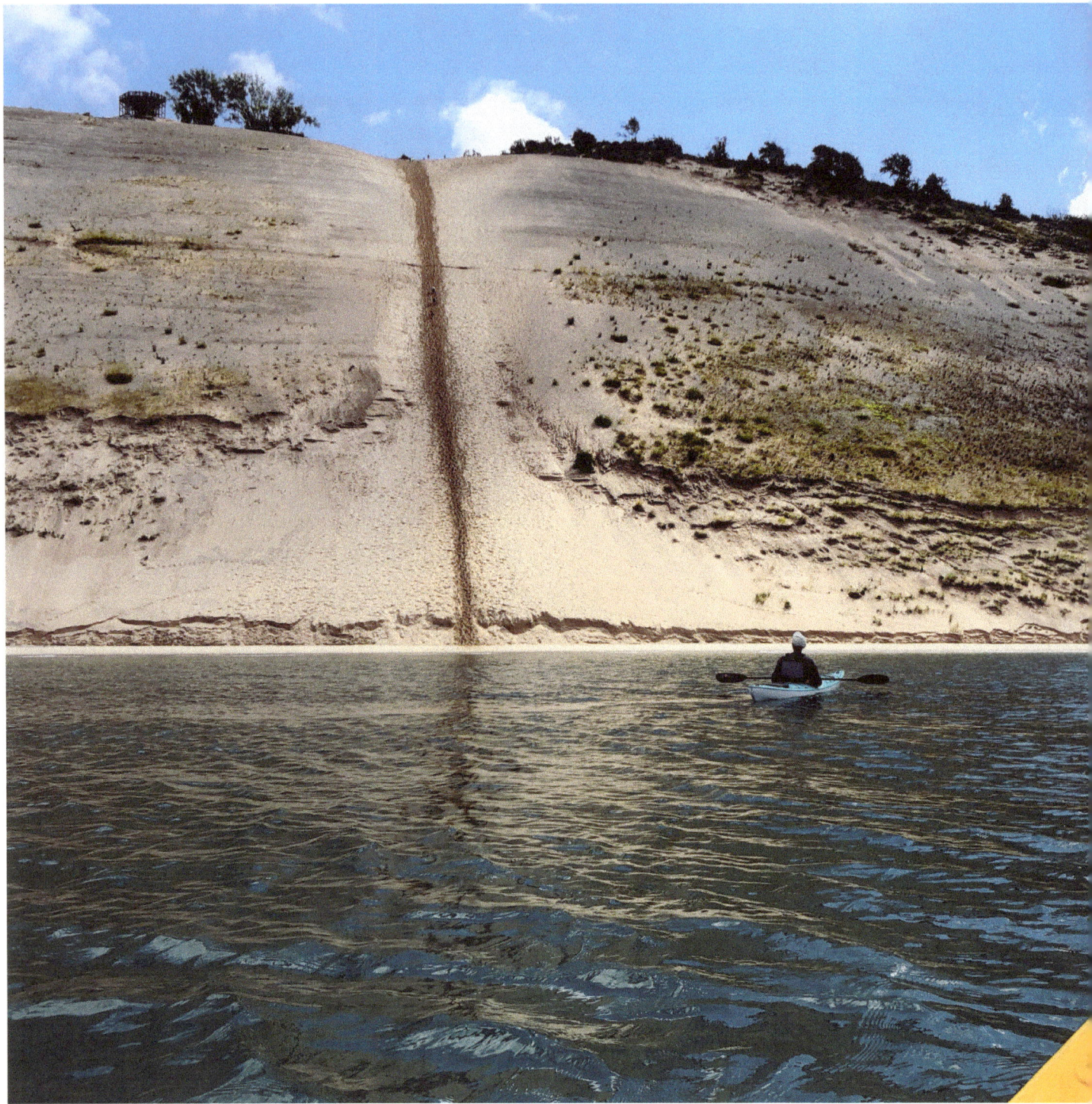

TRIP 2: SLEEPING BEAR DUNES
THE BEAR

For years I visited the Overlook, perched high over the seemingly endless horizon of Lake Michigan, and would often see kayakers paddling in the water way down below. Wouldn't it be fun, I'd say to myself, if I could be down there looking up at the people like me? Eventually I got that chance.

This is my all-time favorite Leelanau paddling location. The experience of paddling on such a big body of water with a wall of sand stretching for miles on one side of your kayak is as good as it ever gets. If you can go when conditions are accommodating, you will have the paddle of a lifetime. We've been fortunate that all three of our paddles to "The Bear" were in the best of conditions.

DATE OF TRIPS: September 26, 2014; August 15, 2016; September 25, 2017; August 30, 2018

LOCATION: Just north of Empire and extending to Glen Haven.

ACCESS: On two of our trips, we put in at the Canning Company parking lot in Glen Haven.

- There is also parking at the Life Saving Station Museum that has access to the lake and is located west of Glen Haven and closer to Sleeping Bear Point.
- From the south, a good access point is the Lake Michigan Beach Park in Empire.
- Another option from the south is the beach at North Bar Lake. The site is off M-22, north of Empire. Take Voice Road west to Bar Lake Road and follow the signs to the parking area. You can also get to the site from Empire by taking LaCore Road north to Voice Road. Turn left onto Bar Lake Road to get to the North Bar Lake parking site. Getting the kayaks to Lake Michigan is a bit more involved here since it requires a longer carry from the parking area and a paddle across North Bar Lake, then another short carry to Lake Michigan. (An option is to carry your kayak on the path around the shoreline of North Bar Lake.) All of these access points have adequate parking and good bathroom facilities. Remember, other than the Empire site, parking requires a National Park pass.

STRATEGIES: If you're using just one vehicle to transport your kayaks, it's important to consider wind direction and wind speeds. The best conditions would be light winds from the east. If you're putting in at Glen Haven, a southerly or easterly wind is preferable. If you are using two vehicles and spotting one, pick the sites that put the prevailing winds to your back as much as possible.

DISTANCE/TIME: The distance from Empire to Glen Haven is approximately 9 miles. It took us about 3 hours of paddling time.

- The distance from Empire to the Pierce Stocking Overlook is approximately 2 miles. It took us about an hour of paddling time.

- The distance from Glen Haven to the Overlook is approximately 5 miles. It took us about 4 hours to do a round trip.

FEATURES:

» The massive sand around the Overlook is an amazing thing to see from a kayak. This wall of sand extends for several miles, from just south of the Overlook, all the way to Sleeping Bear Point. These dunes are called perched sand dunes, or dunes that develop on a pre-existing hill or cliff. Here, the existing cliff is the rock and residue left from the action of the last glacier, about 10,000 years ago. There are also many lower sand dunes as you paddle closer to Glen Haven.

» Landslides of sand are common. There have been several major landslides into Lake Michigan in the last 50 years. Small to medium landslides happen all the time. These give the dunes a very interesting look, one that changes from moment to moment.

» We saw some rare piping plovers on each of our trips. These endangered birds are a protected species, and their nesting areas are well marked by the park rangers.

» Bald eagles and other raptors are very often seen along this stretch of Lake Michigan. In the spring and fall, this is a prime area to watch hawks migrating.

» The Overlook and the Pierce Stocking Trail are two of the most popular features in the National Park. Pierce Stocking (1908-1976) bought land south of Glen Haven from D.H. Day in 1948 and set up a sawmill north of Little Glen Lake. When all the mature trees had been cut, Stocking closed the sawmill and developed a road and a scenic tourist attraction in the dunes.

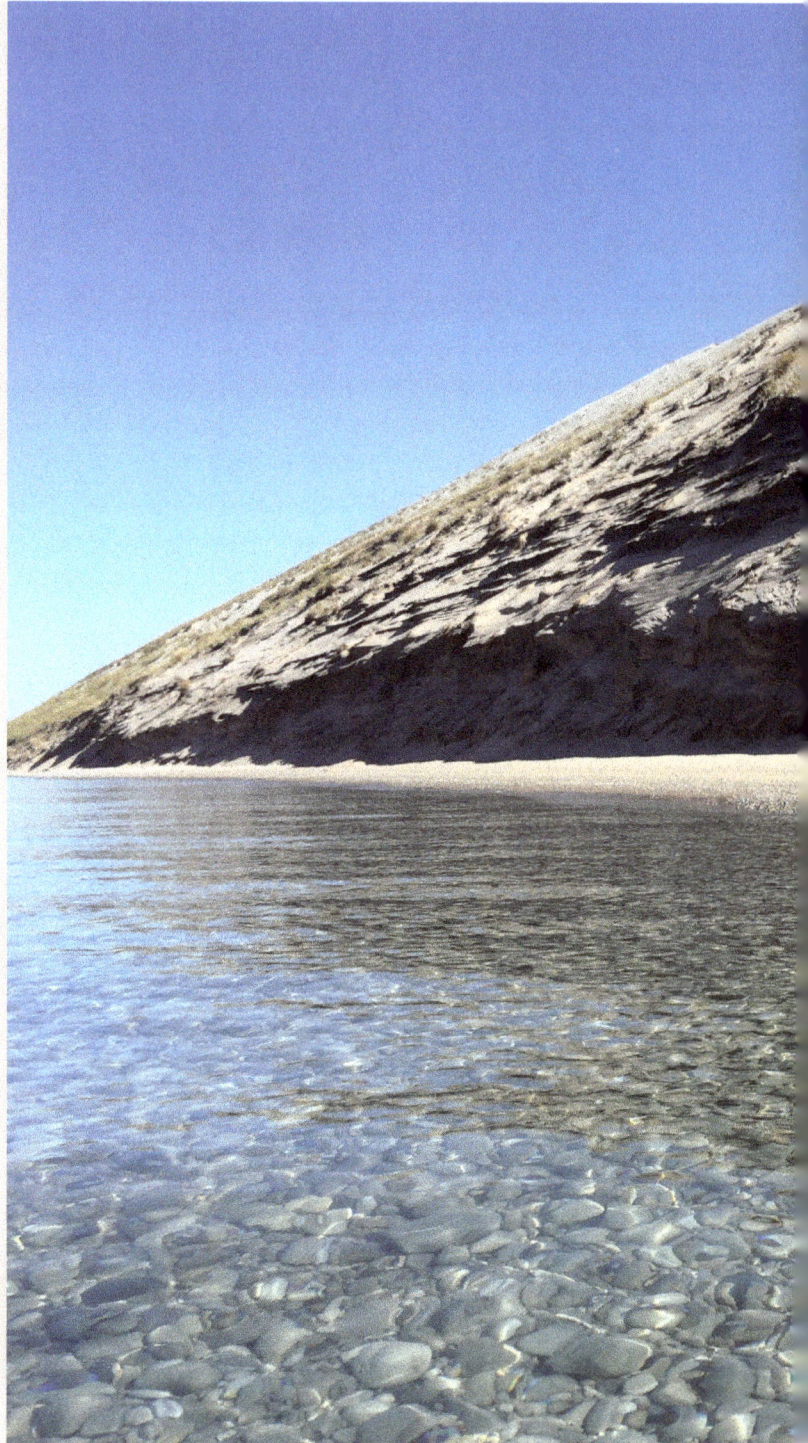

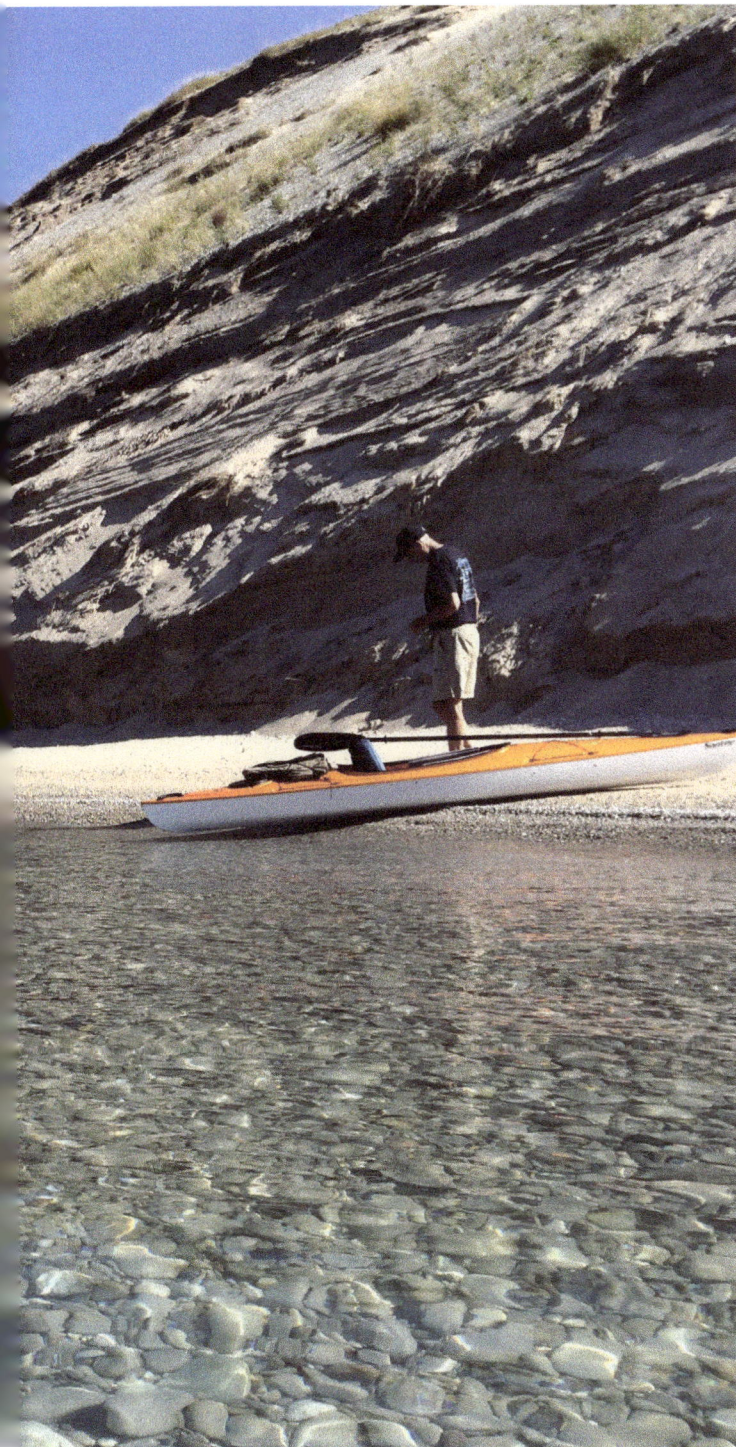

Eventually, that became the Pierce Stocking Trail we enjoy today. The Pierce Stocking Overlook is about 2 miles north of Empire on M-109.

» Sleeping Bear Dunes was authorized as a National Park on October 21, 1970. Senator Philip A. Hart (D-Mich) was instrumental in this action by the Federal government. Today, over one million people visit the park each year.

» We have seen pieces of ships and barges on each of our day trips to Sleeping Bear. There is one wreck (likely it used to be a barge) that is right on the shore near Sleeping Bear Point. These wrecks are reminders of the inherent dangers of Lake Michigan. The National Park Service reminds everyone to leave the shipwrecks alone to let others have the chance to see them.

» The name Sleeping Bear comes from the Ojibwe legend of a huge forest fire on the Wisconsin side of Lake Michigan that drove a mother bear and her two cubs to swim across the lake for safe shelter. The mother bear, upon reaching the shore, waited at the top of a bluff for her cubs. The cubs drowned near shore, but the mother stayed anyway. The Great Spirit was so impressed with the determination of the mother bear that it created the two islands to represent the cubs. They are now called North and South Manitou. Meanwhile, the winds buried the waiting mother under the sands of the dunes, and the "bear" became a tree-covered knoll near the edge of the bluff. Wind and erosion have changed the size and appearance of this "bear" today.

» The Maritime Museum is located just west of Glen Haven. The original life saving station was built in 1901, a little farther west, right on Sleeping Bear Point. The station was moved to its current location in 1931, due to shifting sands and sand slides. There were two methods of rescue: Rescuers could use 23-foot surfboats that rolled on wooden rails to the water or were hauled by horses on a cart down the beach if the rescue was a long distance from the station. The other method was to use a device called a Lyle gun, which shot a line across the deck of a ship and allowed heavier lines to be pulled out to begin rescue procedures.

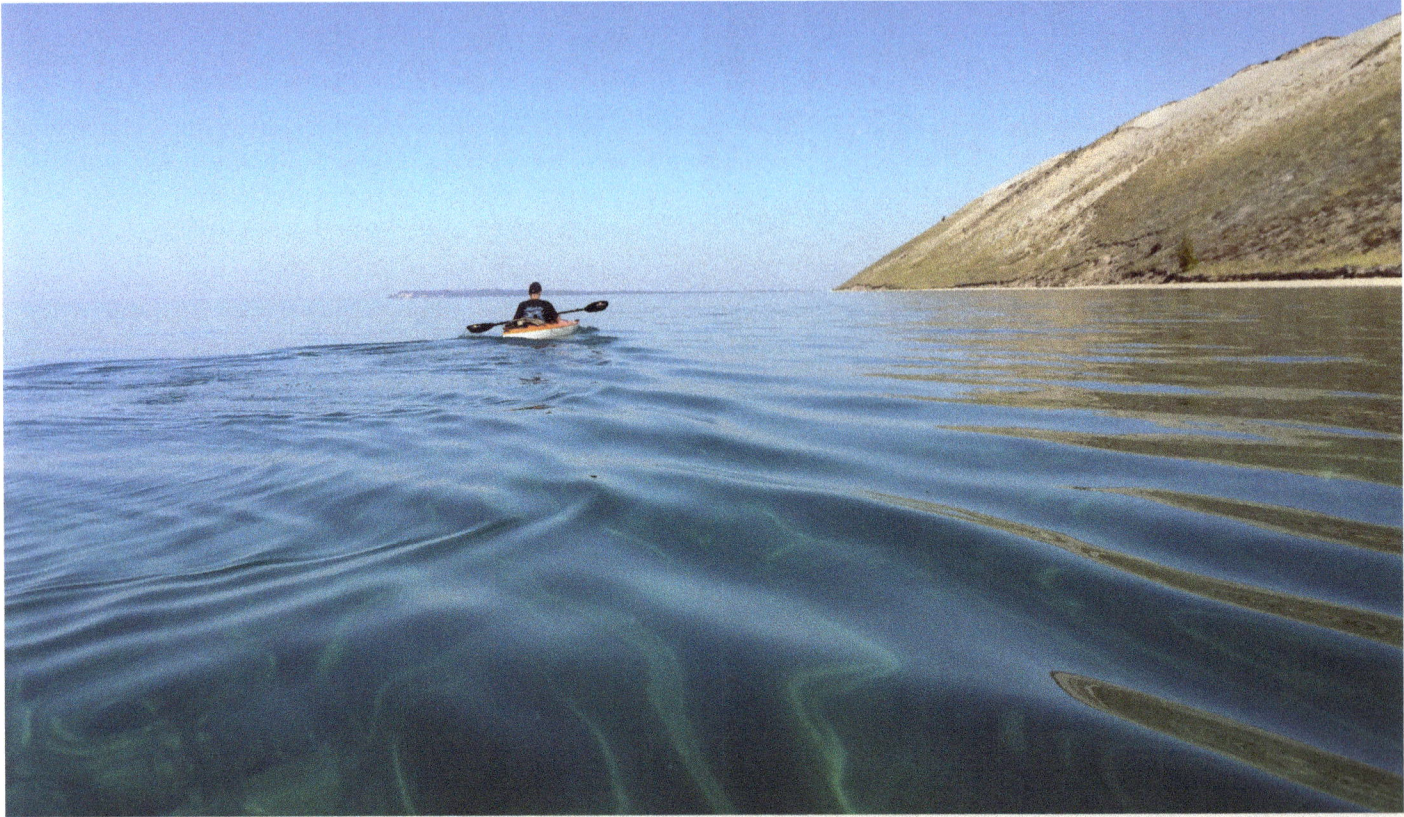

» The Manitou Islands are part of Leelanau County. On this day trip you can get a good view of South Manitou's sandy bluffs and its lighthouse that was built in 1871. The wreck of the *Francisco Morazan* is still visible on the island's southern shore. The ship grounded in 1960 and became a total loss.

» On this trip you are close to the Manitou Passage, one of the most important shipping lanes in the entire Great Lakes, and it's likely that you'll see a deep-draft lake freighter or two. (One interesting tidbit is that President John F. Kennedy's presidential yacht was the "S/Y Manitou," named for the Manitou Passage.) The Manitou Passage has been called the most dangerous passage on the Great Lakes, and is both a mariner's nightmare and a valuable shortcut. There are 50 known shipwrecks in the Passage, and likely many more.

» For years, the most dangerous cargoes to ship were potatoes and Christmas trees. Both had to be shipped late in the shipping season — right at the time when the lakes can have the most ferocious storms.

» During the ice age, the wall of ice would have been 7 to 10 times the height of the huge, sandy dunes of Sleeping Bear — something to consider when looking up at the 450-foot dunes from a kayak in the lake! (Hooker, Thomas H., *The Last Ice Age and the Leelanau*, Dog Ear Press.)

» Sleeping Bear Point used to extend out into Lake Michigan further, creating the "haven" in Glen Haven. With more than 200 acres of sand, it was home to a fishing shanty and the owner's headquarters—until one night in 1915 when the entire point slipped away into the big lake, taking the shanty with it. The remaining sharp bluff that was left behind is now also gone—scoured away by the actions of the wind and water.

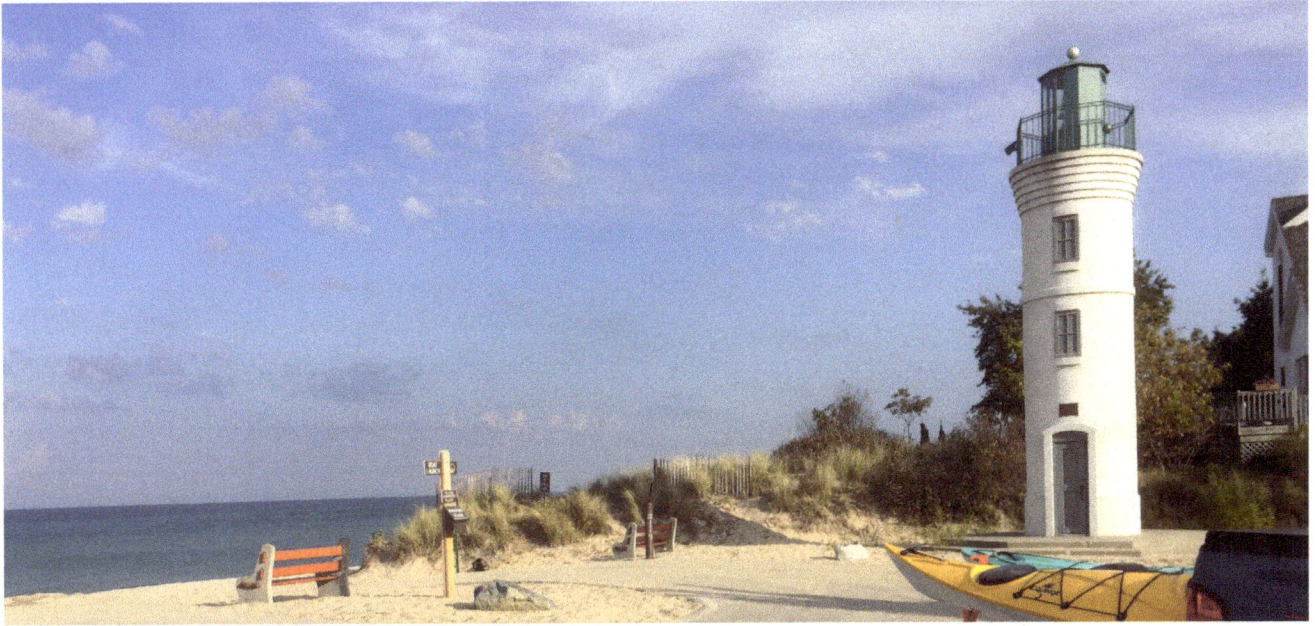

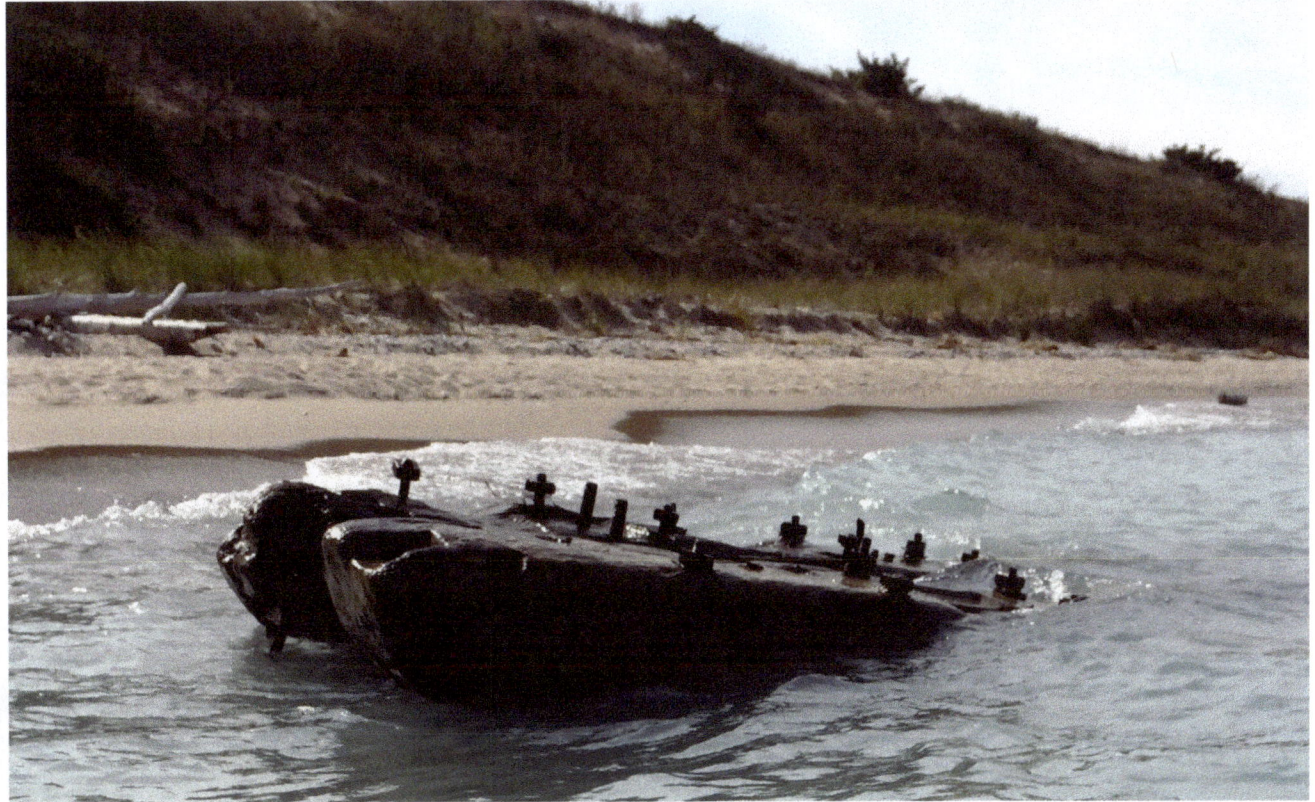

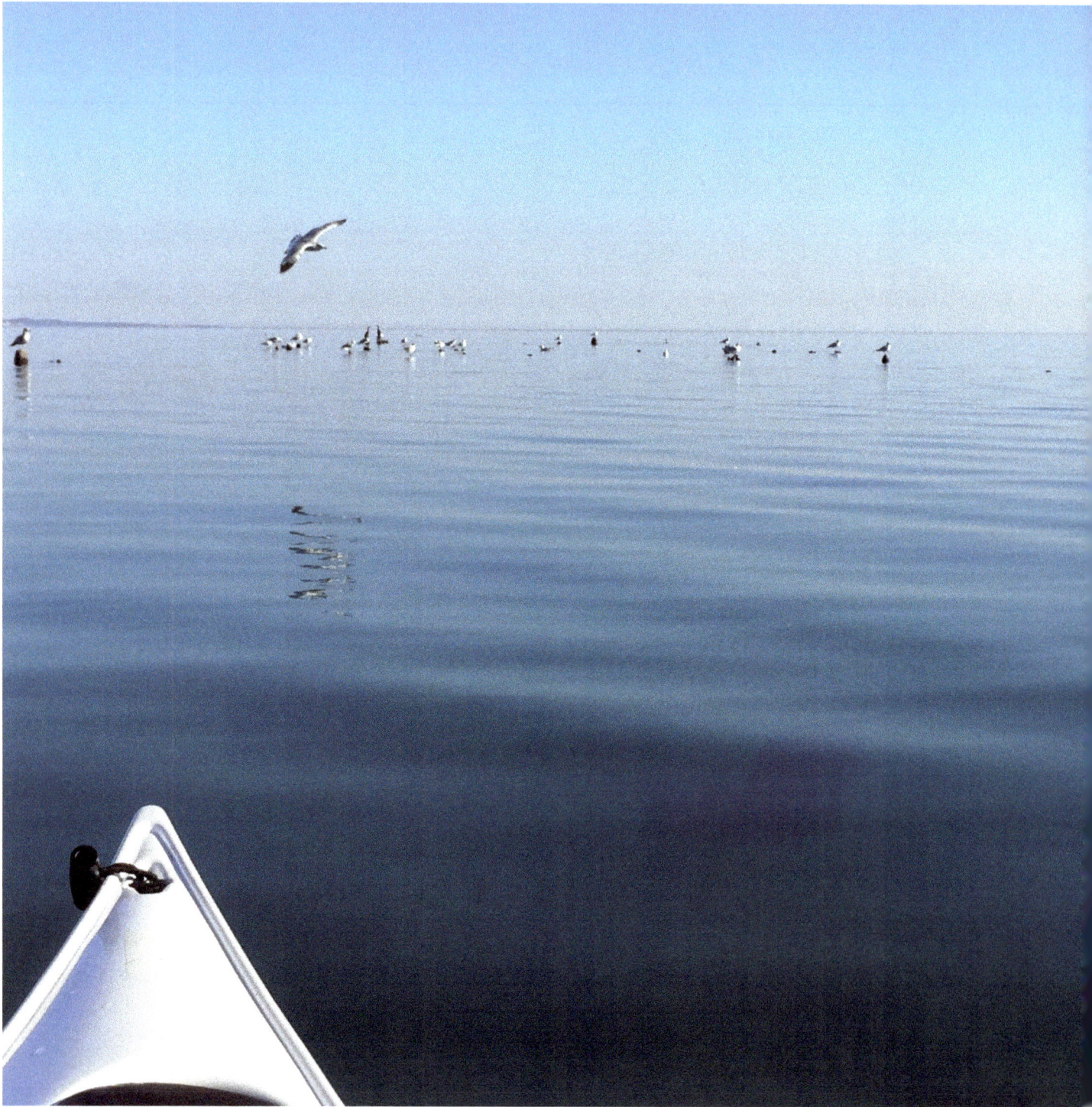

TRIP 3: GLEN HAVEN TO PORT ONEIDA
SLEEPING BEAR BAY

A paddle on Sleeping Bear Bay makes for a great day trip on Lake Michigan. There are such a variety of things to see from a kayak just offshore! The Manitou Islands and the Manitou Passage are to the north. And there's the D.H. Day campsites, many beautiful homes, busy Glen Arbor, the Homestead Resort and miles of quiet areas along the Sleeping Bear National Lakeshore.

This bay is a bit smaller in area and shoreline than Good Harbor Bay further north, but it is just as beautiful.

DATE OF TRIP: August 16, 2017

LOCATION: Glen Haven and Port Oneida.

ACCESS: We launched from Glen Haven at the main beach and parking area near the Canning Building. Bathrooms are available.

- There are other access sites at the ends of roads in Glen Arbor.

- Go north on Lake Street (east of the intersection of M-109 and M-22) or north on Bay Lane (further east on M-22). Park on the street. There are public restrooms in town.

- Our landing site was a beach at the end of a dirt road off Port Oneida Road. (Take M-22 east out of Glen Arbor and turn left on Port Oneida Road.)

- There is also a beach at the end of Lane Road, but access is tricky as there are steep, wooden steps. We had to take one kayak at a time, but we made it just fine.

DISTANCE/TIME: Approximately 7 miles. It took us 2.5 hours to paddle from Glen Haven to Port Oneida with a slight wind at our backs.

FEATURES:

» D. H. Day Campground, located just east of Glen Haven, has 88 private sites and easy access to Lake Michigan. Its address is 8000 W. Harbor Hwy. Glen Arbor, MI 49636.

» Who was D.H. Day? David Henry Day came to Glen Haven in 1878, and was put in charge of the local company that harvested wood and sold it to passing ships for fuel. Eventually, Day borrowed money from Perry Hannah of Traverse City to help buy the Glen Haven operation, a fleet of ships and much of the land in the area. Glen Haven became his Company Town. Day practiced reforestation before it became popular elsewhere. As lumbering declined, he diversified by growing apple and cherry trees, and built the Glen Haven Canning Company on the shoreline near the dock for easy shipping to many Great Lakes cities. He had huge, white barns built just south of Glen Haven in the 1880s for his 400 hogs and prized herd of 200 Holsteins. His barns are now iconic landmarks in the park. In 1920, Day donated 32 acres of his land between Glen Haven and Glen Arbor, which became the D.H. Day State Park (and now part of the National Lakeshore.) D.H. Day died in 1928 at the age of 76.

» Glen Arbor is one of the most popular tourist destinations in Leelanau. It was founded in 1848 as a fueling station for the wood-burning ships on Lake Michigan. It has a population of 788 people, but that number swells tremendously in the summer months.

» The Homestead Resort is a luxurious, four-season resort, with one mile of sandy Lake Michigan shoreline. From the water you can see many of the condos and buildings. There is an interesting development at the mouth of the Crystal River with shops, restaurants and other features.

» The first settler in Port Oneida was Carsten Burfiend in 1852. He was a fisherman, and also ferried people back and forth to the Manitou Islands. He was followed by settlers from Hanover, Germany and Prussia. One of them was Thomas Kelderhouse, who became important in the development of Port Oneida. He built the dock into Lake Michigan. (Port Oneida is named for the SS Oneida, one of the first ships to stop at the dock.) The decline of the lumber industry, the growth of nearby communities and the death of Thomas Kelderhouse in 1884 all contributed to the decline of Port Oneida itself. The cemetery at the intersection of M-22 and Port Oneida Road is called the Kelderhouse Cemetery.

» Port Oneida Rural Historic District was farmed for over 100 years. Consisting of 18 farmsteads, 121 buildings and 3,400 acres, it is the largest historic agricultural community in the U.S. under governmental ownership. The Port Oneida Fair runs on the second Friday and Saturday in August every year.

» A visible feature to the north is the North Manitou Shoal Light, also called "The Crib" (named for the artificial island made of concrete in 21 feet of water). It was built in 1935 to warn ships of the danger of the shallow waters of the North Manitou Shoal Bank that extends 3 miles south from North Manitou Island. The red flashing light is 79 feet above the water and can be seen from 25 miles away.

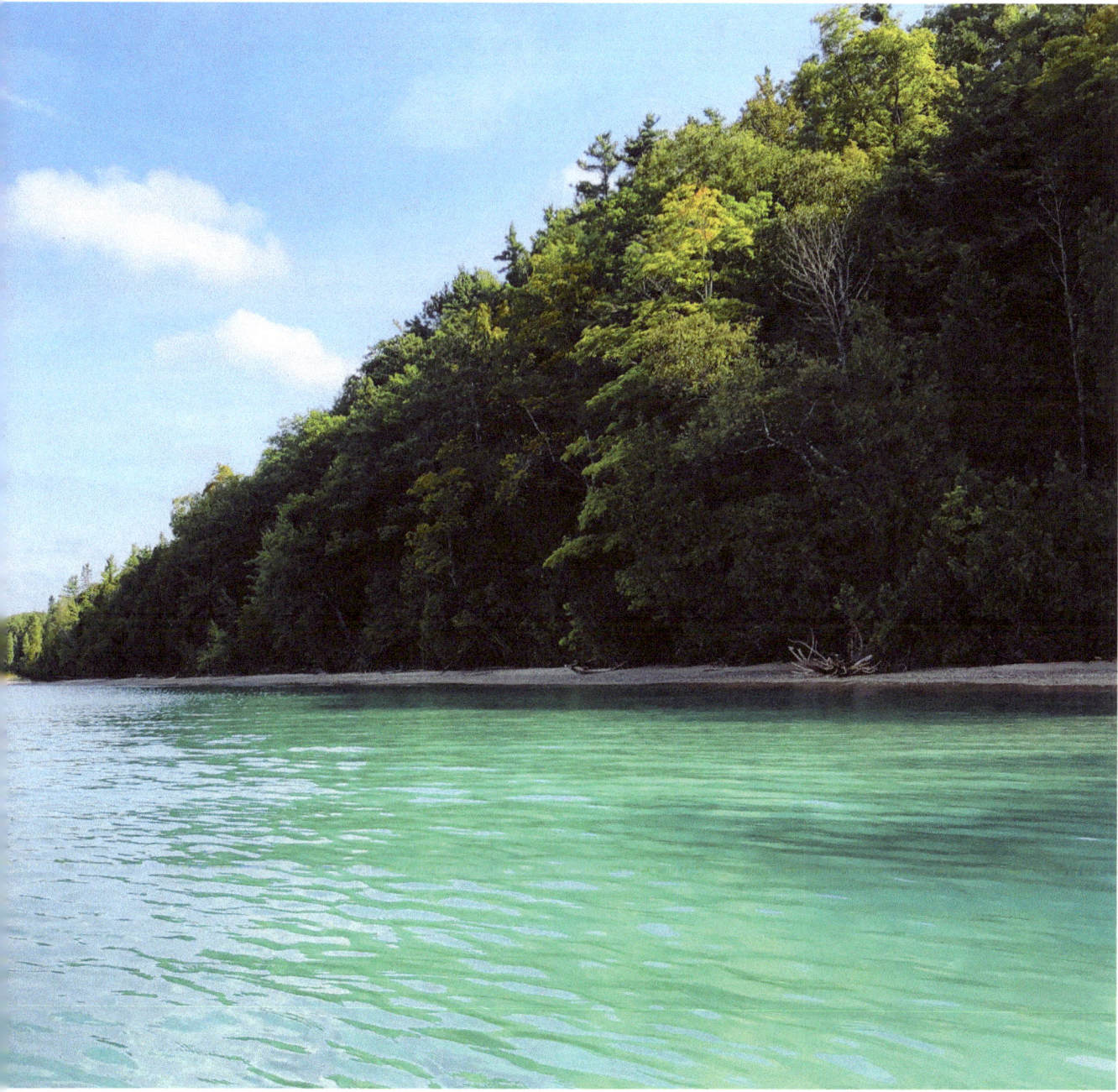

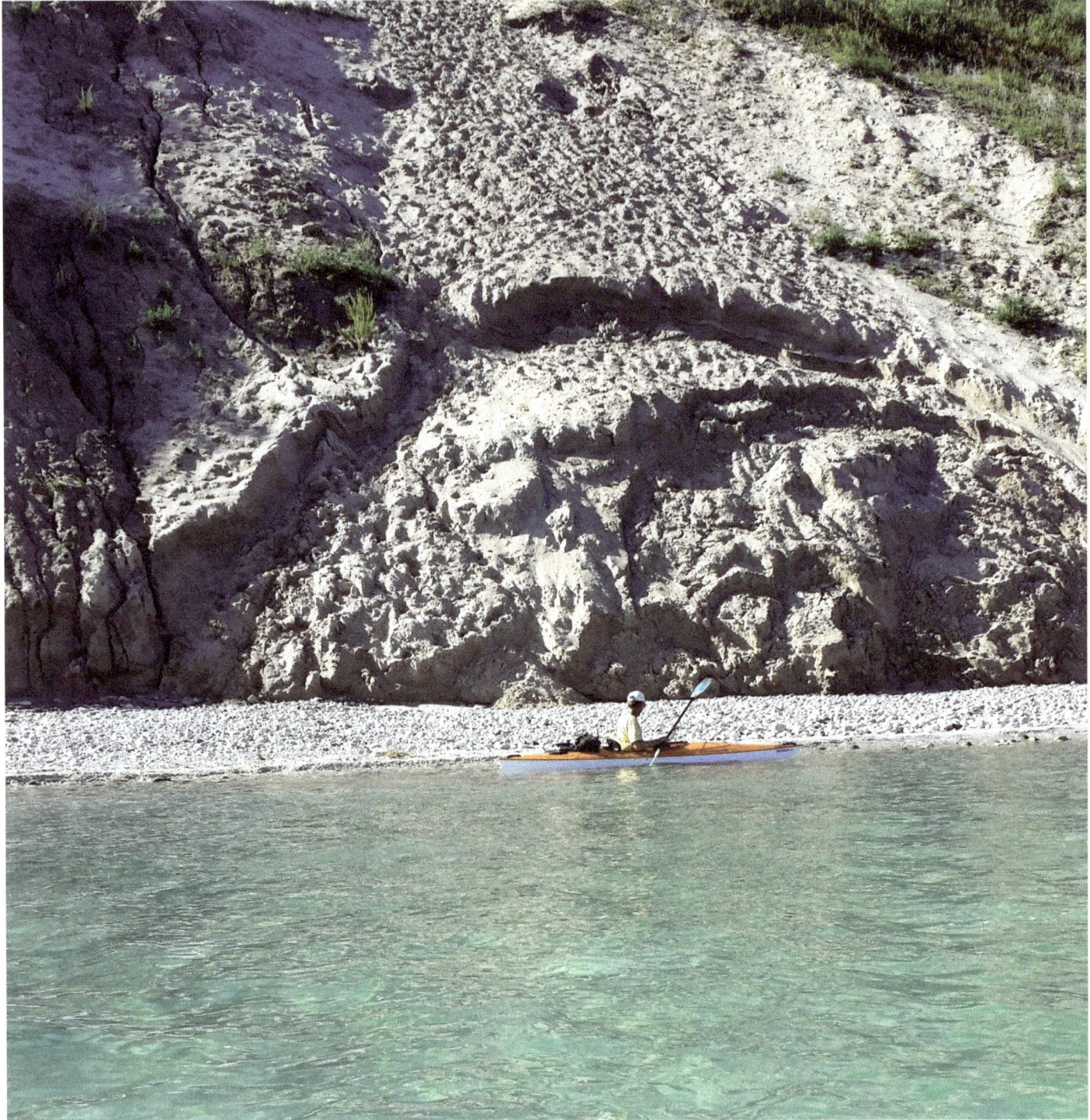

TRIP 4: PORT ONEIDA
TO GOOD HARBOR BEACH
PYRAMID POINT

The highlight of this day trip is paddling by the perched dune at Pyramid Point. The panoramic view from its top takes in both of the Manitou Islands, the Manitou Passage and blue water as far as the horizon. The view from below is dramatic in a different way. Approaching Pyramid Point, you will see much lower ridges with vast expanses of forests right at the edge of the water. Some of the trees have fallen victim to sand slides and erosion. And east of the big dune there is evidence of cottages and other buildings that have also fallen over the edge, due to the erosive action of the winds and the waves of the lake.

Paddling in front of the main perched dune at Pyramid Point is quite different from Sleeping Bear: while it's just as tall or taller, its width is smaller and the mixture of sand and clay give it a different texture. I have been on two trips to Pyramid Point — one with my brother-in-law David Clinton, who joined me during the excellent weather of September 2014, and again with Larry in late August of 2016. Both were exceptionally great day trips. Hopefully, we will be returning to Pyramid Point very soon!

DATE OF TRIPS: September 24, 2014; August 29, 2016; September 24, 2018, August 20, 2019

LOCATION: Pyramid Point separates Sleeping Bear Bay and Good Harbor Bay and is located between Glen Arbor and Leland.

- The hiking trailhead is worth visiting before or after your paddle, and is located about 5 miles northeast of Glen Arbor along M-22. Turn left (north) on Port Oneida Road, which turns into Baesh Road. The trailhead is on the left. The trail itself is a round trip of 1.6 miles up the backside of Pyramid Point Dune. At the lookout, you will be about 370 feet directly above Lake Michigan. The view from the top of Pyramid Point is absolutely amazing. This is one of my favorite views in all of Leelanau!

ACCESS: From the west, the best access point would be the Port Oneida site that we used in trip #3. This is the best option for a two-vehicle strategy.

- From the east, there are several options, the best one being the Sleeping Bear National Lakeshore Beach at the end of Bohemian Road (County Road 669). Parking and restroom facilities are available, and access to the beach is very easy.

- If you want to have a shorter paddle, you can access the water by turning left (west) near the end of Bohemian Road onto Michigan Road (gravel). On Michigan Road, you will be seeing Lake Michigan to your right and also several trails leading directly to the beach. Simply park your vehicle on the roadside and carry your kayak to the shore (about 50 yards).

- If you want a longer paddle on Good Harbor, you can put in at the National Park beach that is located at the end of Good Harbor Trail (County Road 651). Putting in at this location adds about 3.5 miles (one way) to your trip, but the view of this part of Good Harbor Bay and the wooded shoreline north of Little Traverse Lake is worth it.

- I tried to determine the origin of the name "Pyramid Point." The National Park reported that maps from around the Civil War were using the term. Their best guess was that the dune really did look like an Egyptian pyramid to those early sailors.

DISTANCE/TIME: A trip from Port Oneida to the beach at the end of Bohemian Road is approximately 6 miles, and a day trip, one way, and would take about 3 hours.

- A round trip from the beach at the end of Bohemian Road is approximately 7.5 miles, and took us about 3.5 hours.

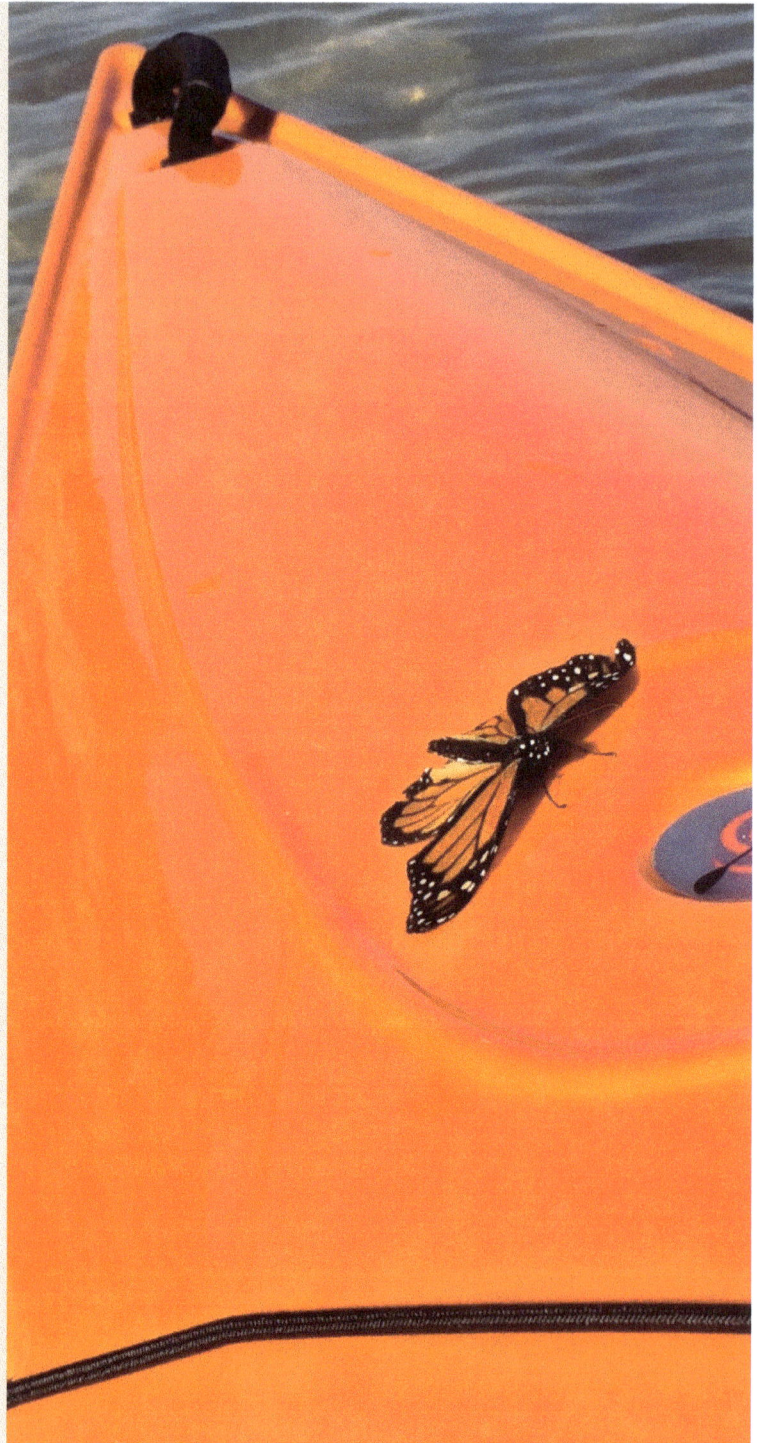

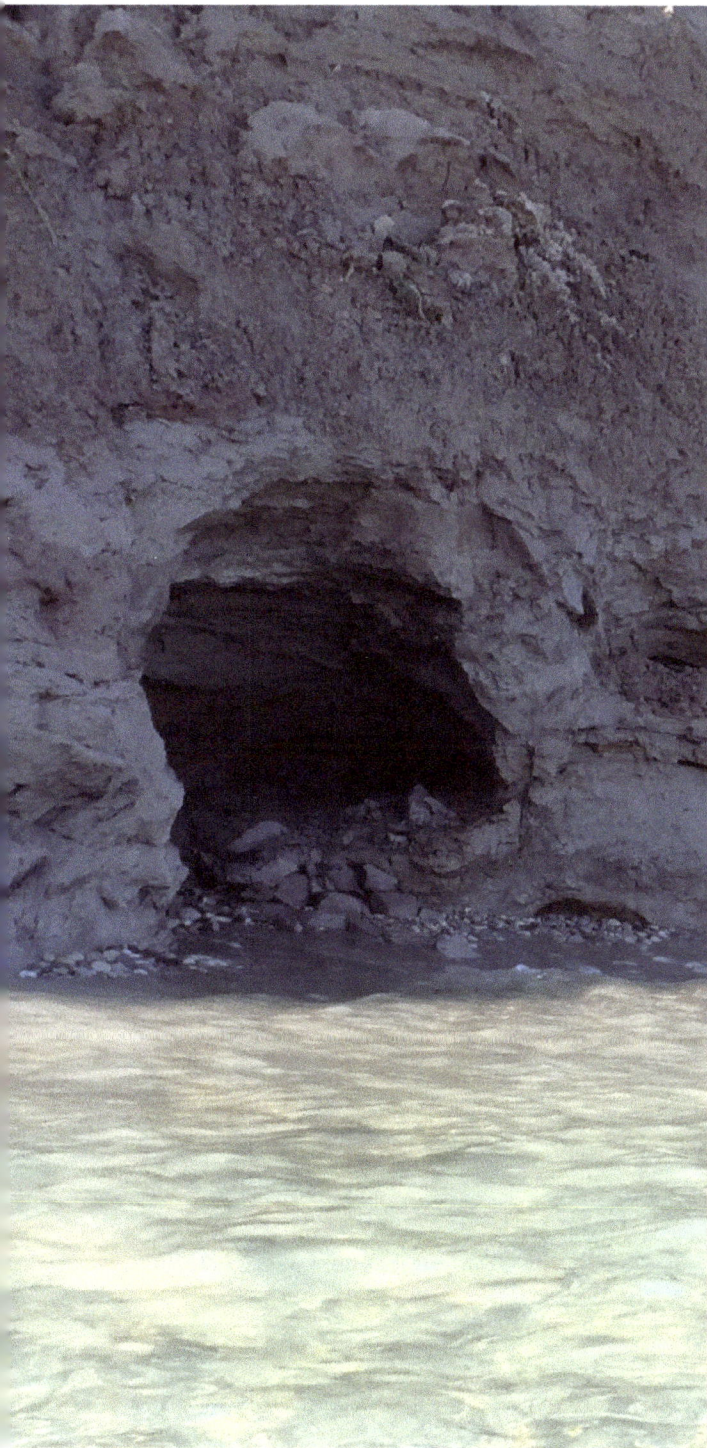

STRATEGIES: The least favorable winds for a trip to Pyramid Point would be from the north or northwest. The most favorable winds would be southwest, south or east.

- If the winds are from the west, you could put in at Port Oneida and have favorable winds at your back to your destination on Good Harbor Bay.

- We had very light winds on both our trips to Pyramid Point.

FEATURES:

» Pyramid Point has been known as a popular spot for hang gliding. I'll stick to kayaking, thank you very much!

» The amount of clay and sand at Pyramid Point makes for very interesting features on the side of the dune. There are markings of many rivulets on the surface of the dune from the rain falling and cascading down the hill.

» One of the things I enjoy about kayaking is that the same area can be quite different each time it's visited. The second time we paddled to Pyramid Point, there were caves in the dune right at the water line. A combination of the higher lake levels, wave action and the clay /sand mixture resulted in this new feature.

» The 133-foot wooden steamer, "The Rising Sun," wrecked just off Pyramid Point in 1917, and the remains are often visible in the shallow waters. Because of variable lake levels, beach erosion, wind and waves, long lost wreck fragments can make unexpected appearances. It's important to remember that these wrecks are considered property of the government and should be viewed but not disturbed.

» On July 27, 2016, during the Chicago Yacht Club race to Mackinac race, the sailboat "The Who Do" sank near the shores of Pyramid Point. It took 12,000 pounds of lift (using airbags) and three hours to bring the 19,000-pound boat up so it could be towed to Charlevoix.

» One of the ghost towns of Leelanau was North Unity (Shalda Corners), located at the spot where Shalda Creek enters Good Harbor Bay and Lake Michigan. The first settler was Frank Kraitz from Bohemia, via Chicago — a typhoid epidemic in Chicago caused the Kraitz family and their Czech friends to look for other places on Lake Michigan to settle. In a scene reminiscent of the Pilgrims, the first winter at North Unity was dreadful, and the little community was near starvation. Frank Kraitz and a few men walked across the ice to North Manitou Island and were able to buy a few bushels of potatoes, which they hauled back across the Manitou Passage on a sled. The men barely made it as the ice was cracking and breaking apart as they neared home. Soon, the village thrived as more people arrived and a schoolhouse, a sawmill, a store, a gristmill and more homes were built. North Unity was granted a post office in 1859. In 1871, a fire broke out on the same day and time as the Great Chicago Fire and the Peshtigo fire in Wisconsin. The fire destroyed North Unity, and the families moved inland to Shalda Corners, at the intersection of M-22 and County Road 669. There is no evidence today of North Unity, but there are some cabins and other structures remaining from Shalda Corners.

» In the fall, this area is an important resting destination for birds and butterflies crossing Lake Michigan. On the 2014 trip, my brother-in-law and I were watching some monarch butterflies arrive from the Upper Peninsula across the open water of Lake Michigan. When one fell from the sky and landed next to my kayak, I scooped him up with my paddle and set him carefully on the bow of my boat. After a little rest, it took off and continued its journey to Mexico. All in a day's paddle.

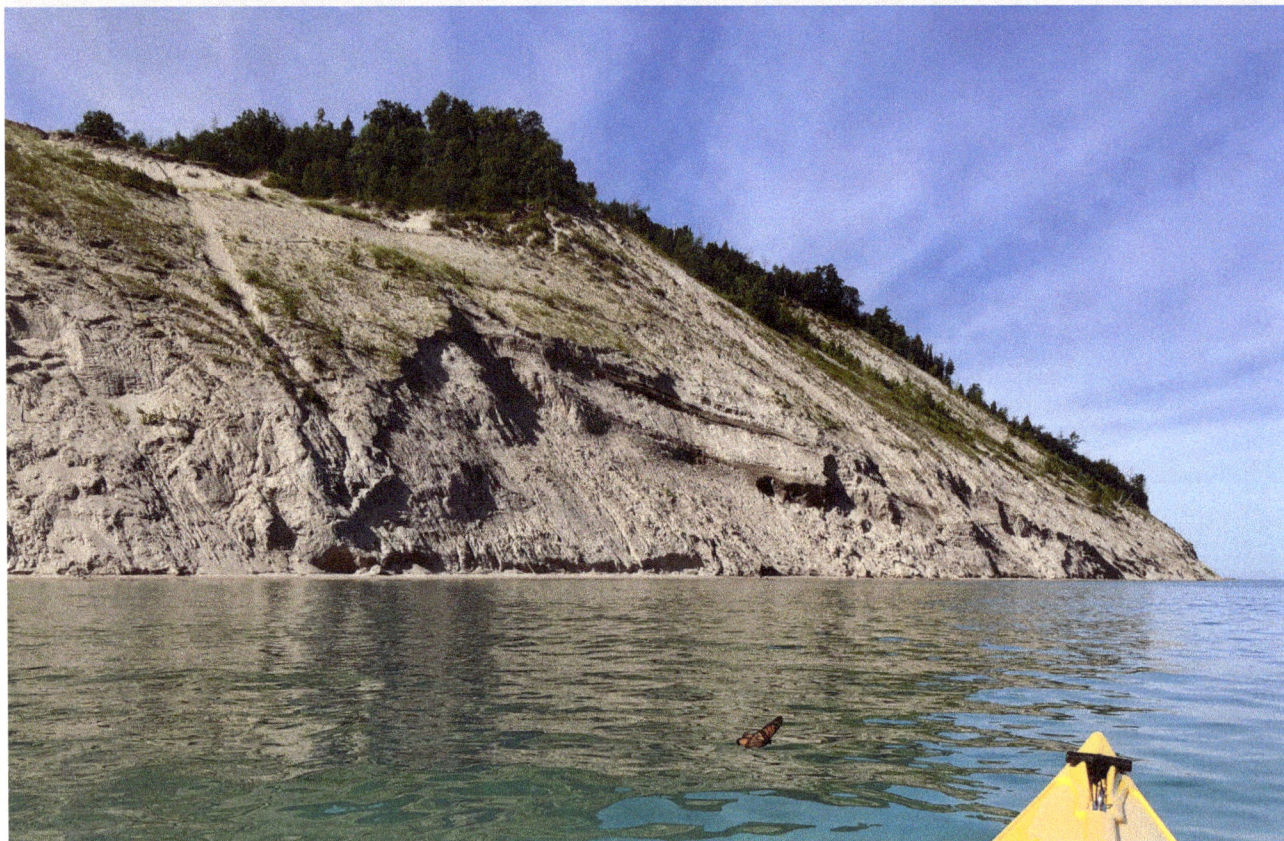

FERRY ROUTE TO LELAND

North Manitou

MANITOU PASSAGE

MAIN SHIPPING LANE

BUOY 6

Pyramid Point Shoal

Turning Point

BUOY 5

Good Harbor Bay

Pyramid Point

Port Oneida

Sleeping Bear Dunes

Shell Lake

National

Lakeshore

Lake Michigan

Narada Lake

22

Bass Lake

School Lake

22

Sleeping Bear Bay

Shown at a larger scale on Plate 4.

Glen Haven

22

SLEEPING BEAR DUNES
NATIONAL LAKESHORE

Glen Arbor

ng Bear
nt

To Grand

shoal Light ("rib")

turning red light

45°00'

44°55'

669

PLATE 5

230 19 43 37 205 274 240
163 30 115 26 89 149 176 260 250
57 41 58 184 150 174 53 231
65 30 19 170 140 197 60 50 68 215 226 221
265 40 114 145 156 176 185 163 160 38 44 45°00'
259 44 130 103 35 36 40 17 19 185
71 60 40 136 32 20 30
297 114 59 48 114 118 135 146 18 25 12 17 142 152
301 262 204 155 124 61 127 25 23 21 17 21 25
306 290 175 86 38 7 15 21 27 112
310 295 54 29 21 21 24
307 260 52 12 10 21
305 292 225 181 147 29 20 10
284 235 180 38 18
298 278 263 196 39 12
247 250 123 37 11 18 4 3
230 275 139 4 3
229 270 280 2
180 157 230 15 4
170 244 150 75 8
79 35 75
60 107
80 90
30 30
10

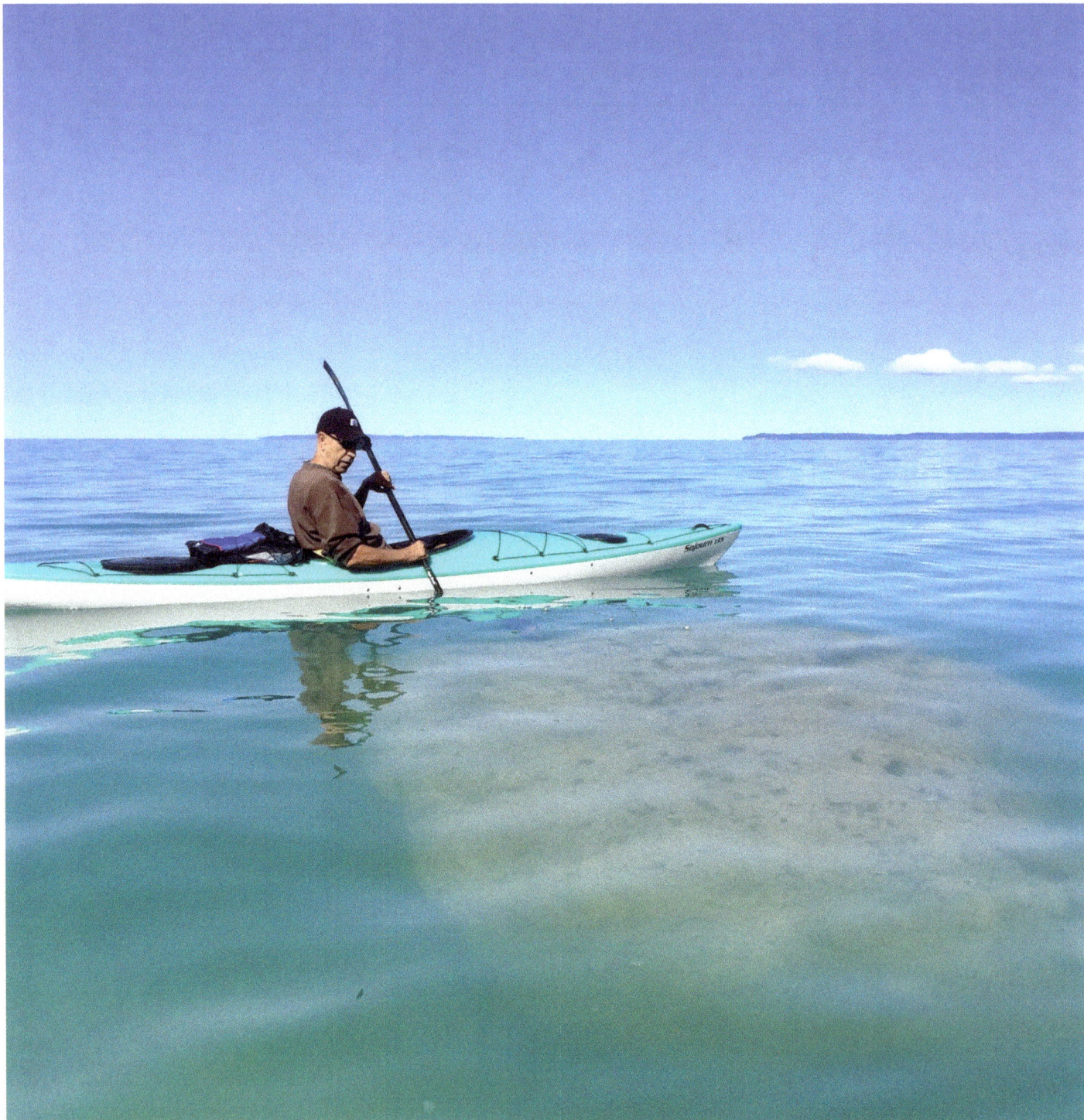

TRIP 5: GOOD HARBOR BAY FROM LELAND

This trip is in the heart of Leelanau — sandy beaches, a view of Sugarloaf Mountain, beautiful water, some higher bluffs near Leland and Leland itself with its harbor and Fishtown.

Because of Good Harbor Bay's relatively shallow and clear water, you can see the rocks and sand formations on the bottom. On the day we paddled here, we noticed the results of recent big waves on the sandy bottom. The many ridges and lines were very interesting.

DATE OF TRIP: August 25, 2017

LOCATION: Leland is midway up the western shore of Leelanau County, at the mouth of the Leland River. The Leland River (also known as Carp River) flows out of beautiful North Lake Leelanau, past Fishtown and the Leland Marina to Lake Michigan.

- Good Harbor Bay is the largest bay on the Leelanau Peninsula, and is located between Pyramid Point and Carp River Point. Good Harbor Bay is 11 miles of the prettiest shoreline in the Great Lakes. Much of the shore is protected land that is part of the Sleeping Bear Dunes National Lakeshore. M-22 runs along its southern edge.

ACCESS: There are several access points in and around Leland.

- Van's Beach: A local favorite located just beyond Van's Garage at the end of Cedar Street. There are portable toilets and some parking — if you get there early. If you don't, there is parking on nearby streets.

- South Beach (Christmas Tree Cove): Public access to Lake Michigan is at the end of Reynolds Street, just west of Main Street.

- North Beach: This beach is located north of the Leland Harbor, off North Lake Street at William Street.

- The access points along Good Harbor include the two beaches in the National Lakeshore. We used the one nearer to Leland at the end of Good Harbor Trail (County Road 651). The other access is the beach at the end of Bohemian Road (County Road 669).

DISTANCE/TIME: Our trip from Van's Beach in Leland to the closer Good Harbor beach at the end of Good Harbor Trail was about 5 miles and took us about 2.15 hours. There was just the slightest of wind that day from the west.

STRATEGIES: Easterly would be the best winds for a day trip here, which although not common, do occur. Be wary of strong winds from any other direction as there is open water from three directions. Lighter winds from the north or south would be deciding factors of which direction to paddle if you are using two vehicles.

FEATURES:

» Just south of Leland there is a big bluff known as Whaleback, rising about 300 feet above Carp River Point and Lake Michigan. This bluff is what geologists call a moraine or drumlin. It was built by the glaciers 10,000 years ago from deposits, and formed into a giant oval by the action of the ice. From the water, the emerald green trees give it a sharp contrast with the blue hues of the water. Whaleback reminds me of Diamondhead in Honolulu, Hawaii.

» Leland was the site of one of the oldest and largest Ottawa villages in the area. There was a natural fish ladder where the dam is now, and the area was an important fishing grounds. Europeans began arriving in the 1830s, also attracted by the abundance of fish. A sawmill was built on the river in 1854, the same year as the first dam. Wooden docks were extended into Lake Michigan, which allowed schooners, and eventually steam ships, to transport settlers and supplies. From 1870 to 1884 the Leland Lake Superior Iron Company ran an iron smelter just north of the mouth of the river. The ore came from the Upper Peninsula, and the charcoal to power the plant came from local timber. The operation produced 40 tons of iron per day. When the iron plant was sold, a sawmill and shingle mill operated from 1885–1900. Around 1900, very wealthy families from Chicago, Cincinnati, Indianapolis and other Midwest cities began building summer cottages, leading to Leland becoming the resort and tourist destination it is today.

» Leland Blue Stones, found along the shore, are a beautiful reminder of Leland's past. These "stones" are slag from the long-gone Leland Iron Works, polished by the waves and sand over many years. Beautiful jewelry is made from these unique "gems."

» The beachfront property south of Leland along M-22 is some of the most desired property in Leelanau County. The views and the sunsets here are amazing. Paddling along the shore in front of these homes and cottages allows the kayaker a glimpse of these fantastic properties. The grand architecture along the shore gives way to the sweeping beauty of the Sleeping Bear National Lakeshore. Here, there are no buildings or expensive landscaping — just the serenity and grandeur of nature. Both of these have their place in this section of Leelanau.

» Once a thriving lumber town, Good Harbor was located at the end of County Road 651 — our destination on this trip. The first dock was built in 1863, with trees cut between Lime and Little Traverse Lakes. The logs were then floated across Little Traverse Lake on a scow pulled by a cable, then transported by tramway to the Lake Michigan shore. The village of Good Harbor was founded a little later, in the mid-1870s, and eventually grew into a large lumber and shipping operation. A new, 500-foot dock was built so that four schooners could be loaded at the same time. Forest products and agricultural goods, like locally grown potatoes, were the main products. The village boasted a hotel, two stores, houses, a school and a saloon. Because of a township line running right down the middle of Main Street, Good Harbor's drinking establishment had to be built on the right side of the street to avoid the rival township's ban on saloons. Eventually, the supply of timber ran out and fires destroyed several of the buildings. The harbor also had little protection from north and northwest storms, and schooners would have to leave the docks for the protection of the Manitou Islands when heavy winds approached. Sometimes, they didn't have time, and the boats were damaged or destroyed. By 1907, the village buildings were torn down and Good Harbor was no more. The only evidence of the village is a few dock pilings in and near the shore.

» When we launched from Vann's Beach, I noticed that the transit boat to South Manitou Island was also leaving Leland. Back in the 1980s, when Larry was my JV Basketball coach, I thought it would be great fun to have him and the rest of my staff (Tom Kozelko and Jerry Schreiner) take that boat out to South Manitou for a "staff bonding" experience. Unfortunately, the wind and waves that day were very strong, resulting in a serious case of sea sickness for two of us. (Not to mention any names, but Tom and I did great.) The highlight of our visit to the island was climbing the spiral staircase to the top of the lighthouse, walking out on the platforms and getting blasted by 40 mile an hour winds. Of course, we had to face the same waves and wind on our trip back, and the same two got sick again. Some great bonding experience. It's a story that never grows old when we get together. And, if you see a photo of Larry paddling with the Leland Manitou in the background, you'll know why he has that pained look on his face.

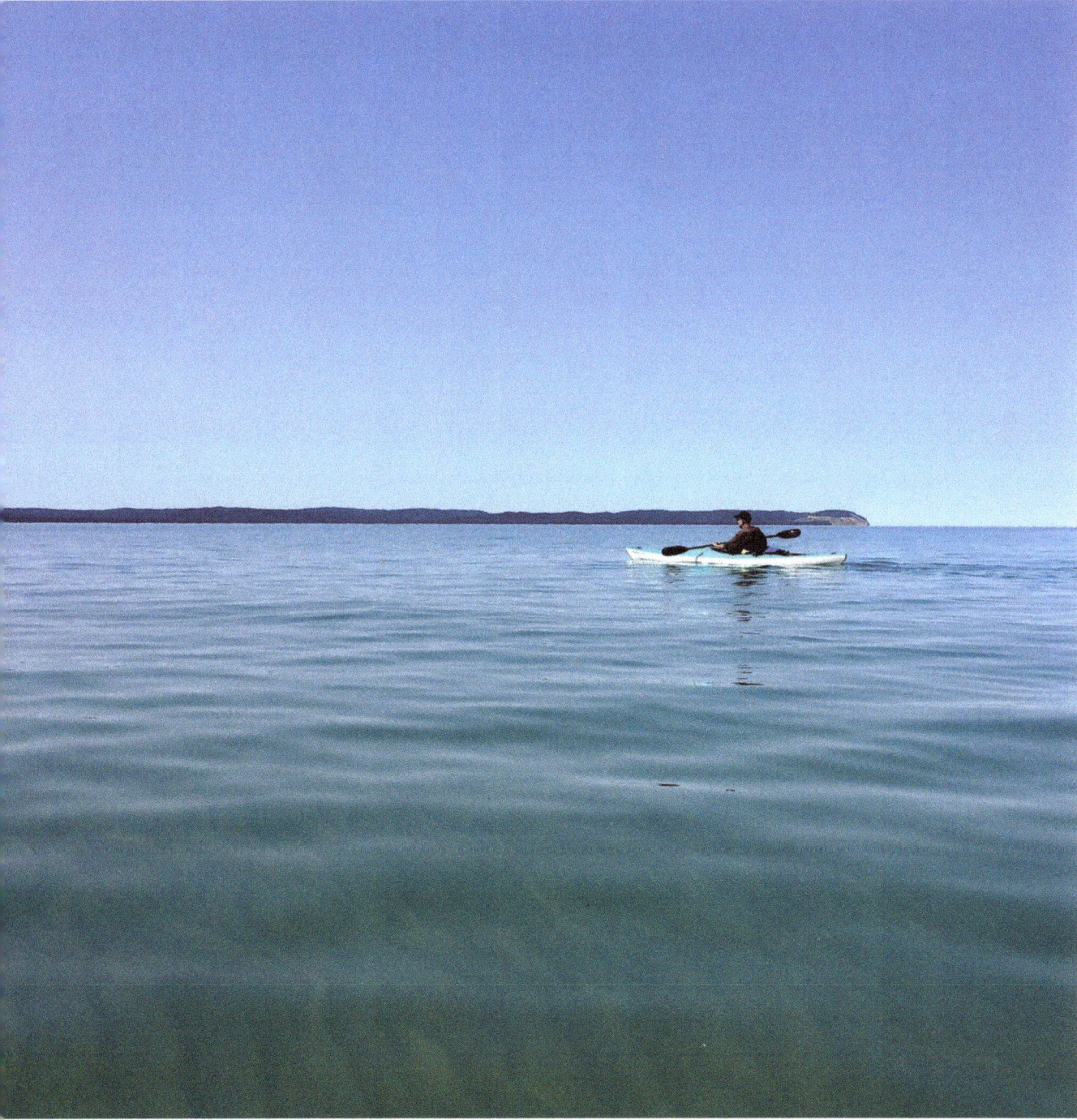

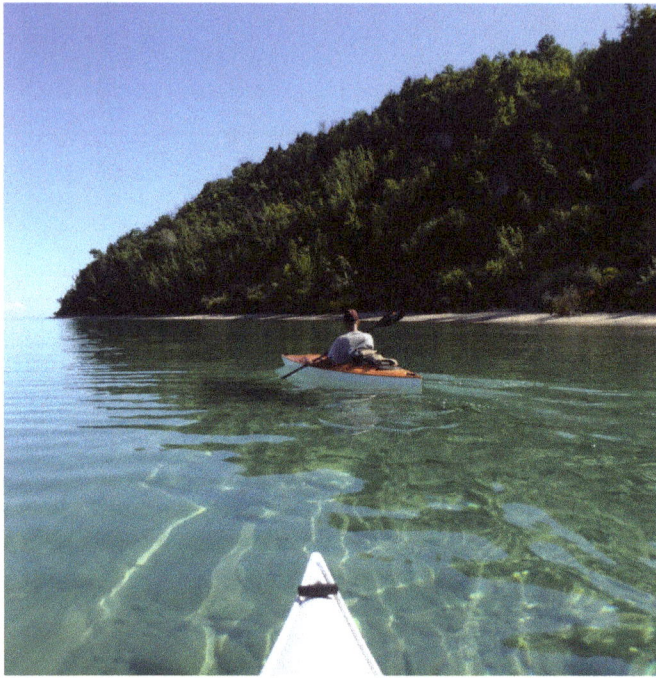
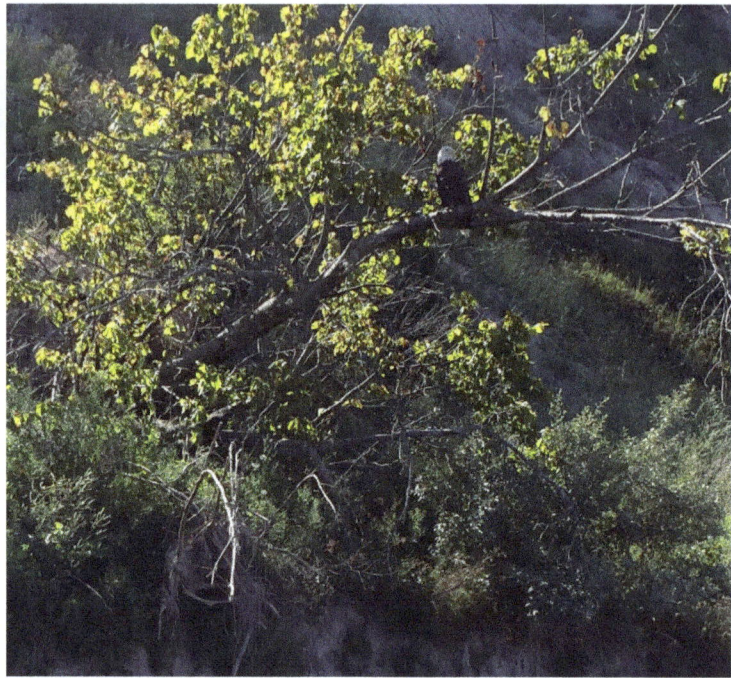
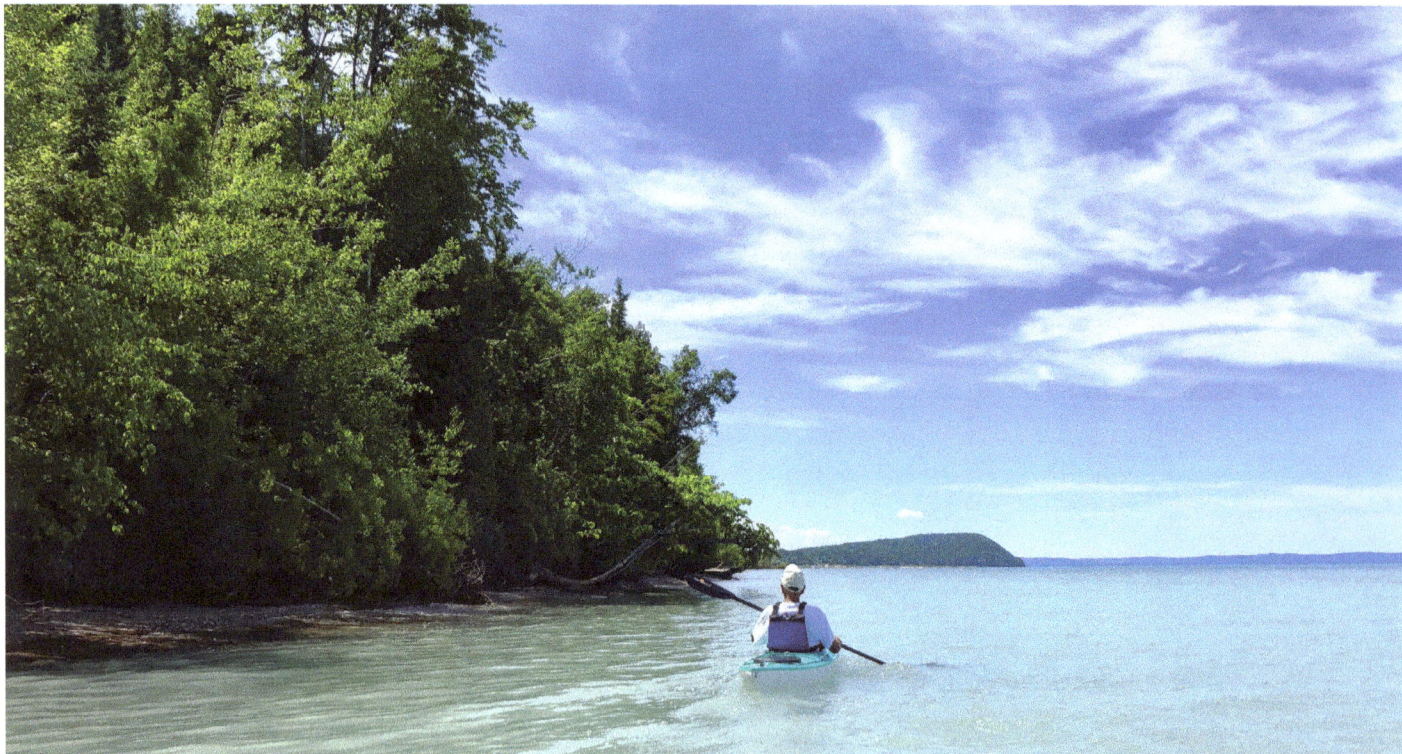

TRIP 6: LELAND AND NORTH TO THE CLAY CLIFFS

This day-trip turned into one of the most pleasant surprises of all our times paddling off the coast of Leelanau. Other areas, like the Sleeping Bear Dunes and Pyramid Point, are much better known and get more visitors, but the colors of the water, sky and wooded shoreline were as good as it gets for kayaking — and for observing nature's beauty.

DATE OF TRIPS: August 8, 2016 and July 10, 2018

LOCATION: The Leland Clay Cliffs are located a little more than one mile north of Leland. The cliffs are tucked between North Lake Leelanau and Lake Michigan.

ACCESS: We used the same Vann's Beach in Leland that was our access point on the previous trip. We used one vehicle and made a round trip. On our second trip on this section in 2018 we started at the beach at the end of Onomonee Road which is located north of M-22 between Leland and Northport. The road and beach can be reached by taking Gills Pier Road, which is located directly across from the location of Fischer's Happy Hour Tavern on M-22. Go north to Onomonee Road and turn left to access the beach at the end of the road.

- The nearest access point north that I know of is Gills Pier, at the beach at the end of Onomonee Road.

DISTANCE/TIME: The distance to the main area of the Leland Clay Cliffs from Vann's Beach is approximately 1.5 miles. It took us about 3 hours to paddle from Leland, past the Clay Cliffs, to Gills Pier and back.

- The distance via water from Leland to the access point at the end of Onomonee Road is approximately 7.5 miles.

STRATEGIES: This area's exposure to winds from the west, northwest and north means that care must be taken on when to go and which way to paddle. Calm conditions or light winds from the south or east are optimal.

- We used a two vehicle strategy on our second visit. We paddled southwest going from Onomonee Road to Vann's Beach in Leland. The trip took us 3 hours in calm, near perfect conditions on Lake Michigan.

FEATURES:

» Leland's Fishtown is a tourist tradition. This historic group of weathered shanties and buildings, many built in the 1800s, now house shops, smokehouses, eateries and other attractions. My personal favorite is the Cheese House — try a tasty sandwich after a day paddling on the water. Commercial fishing here began around 1880, and eventually as many as eight fishing tugs ventured out on the Big Lake in search of whitefish, trout and other fish. Today, two fish tugs, the *Joy* and the *Janice Sue*, continue that tradition. For more than a century, the Carlson family has operated a fishery here. Nels Carlson emigrated from Norway and began the operation, the present Nels Carlson is the fifth generation to keep the fishery going.

» Leland Township Marina is right next to Fishtown, and one of the most popular marinas on Lake Michigan. It has 45 slips and one commercial slip. Leland Harbor is a Harbor of Refuge, which means boats must be accepted even if they have to be tied together in the protection of the harbor.

» Because of the shoaling of sand near the entrance of the marina, dredging is an annual need. As a way to find a long term funding solution to the costs, the community and others raised money to purchase a 28-ton dredge on April 7, 2017.

» The Clay Cliffs have their own unique look. Rugged and worn by the actions of wind and water, the area makes for excellent viewing from the cockpit of a kayak. These bluffs rise almost vertically over 200 feet above the shore. In 2013, the Leland Clay Cliffs area was designated a Leland Township natural area to be managed by the Leelanau Land Conservancy. Some homes remain, however, that are outside the protected Conservancy land, and several of them are endangered by landslides and erosion. Many of the owners have built intricate wooden stairways to the shore, and some of them have been destroyed or damaged by the power of nature.

» The unique topography and micro-climate of this area have created one of the most rare and fragile wildflower habitats in northern Michigan. Trillium, dutchman's breeches, doll's eyes, and many other native flowers are found here.

» This area is known for its bald eagles. We saw a nesting pair and one of their fledglings on our paddle. They were watching us, too.

» There is a 1.6-mile hiking trail to view the Leland Clay Cliffs from above. The trailhead is located just north of Leland, along M-22.

» One of the more unique experiences on this trip occurred when we got to Vann's Beach and were transporting our kayaks to the water. We noticed that we were not completely alone: there was a lady doing yoga and a young man playing a flute. No doubt because sound travels so well over water, we were able to enjoy the haunting notes long into our paddle. A very unique moment, indeed.

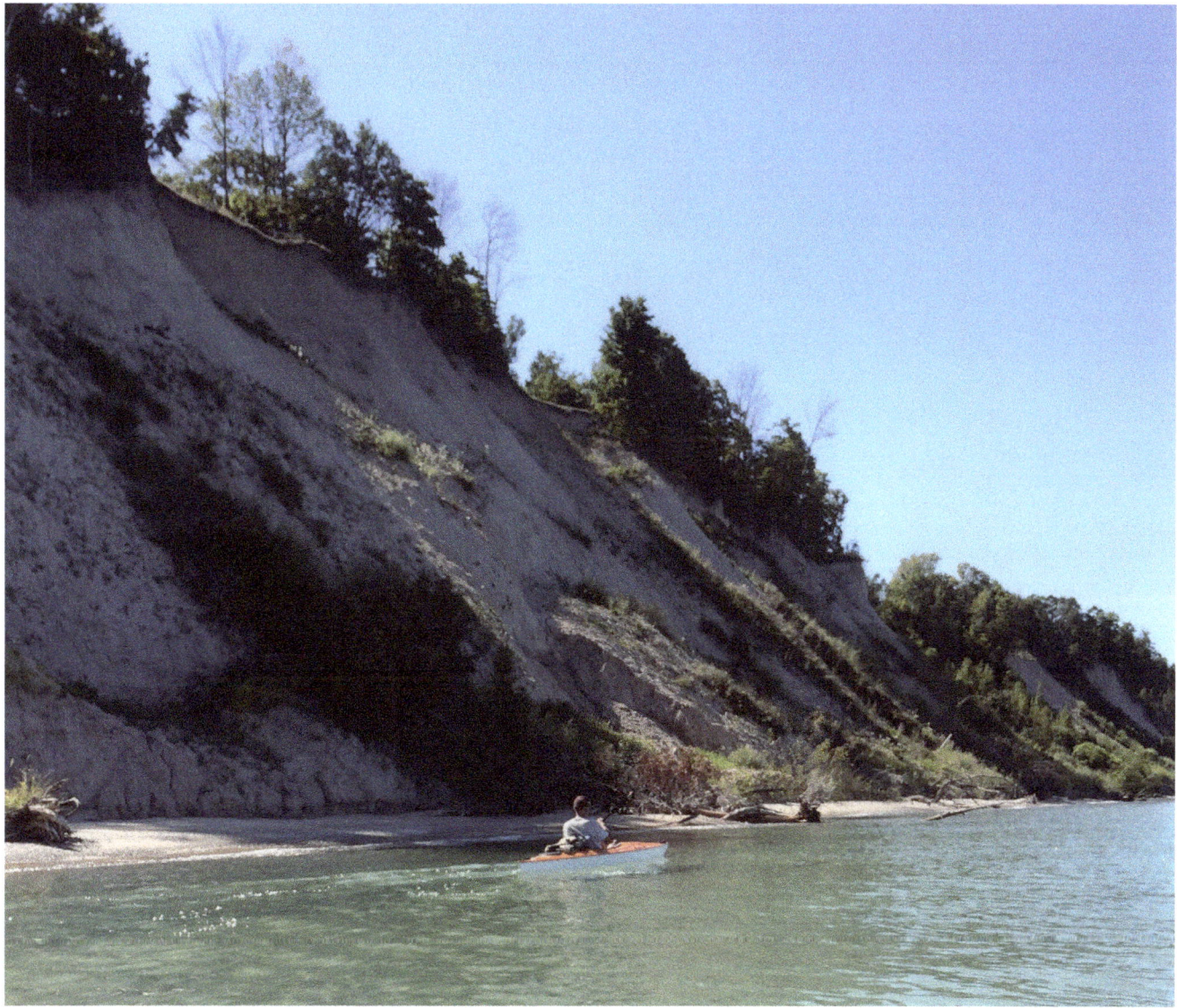

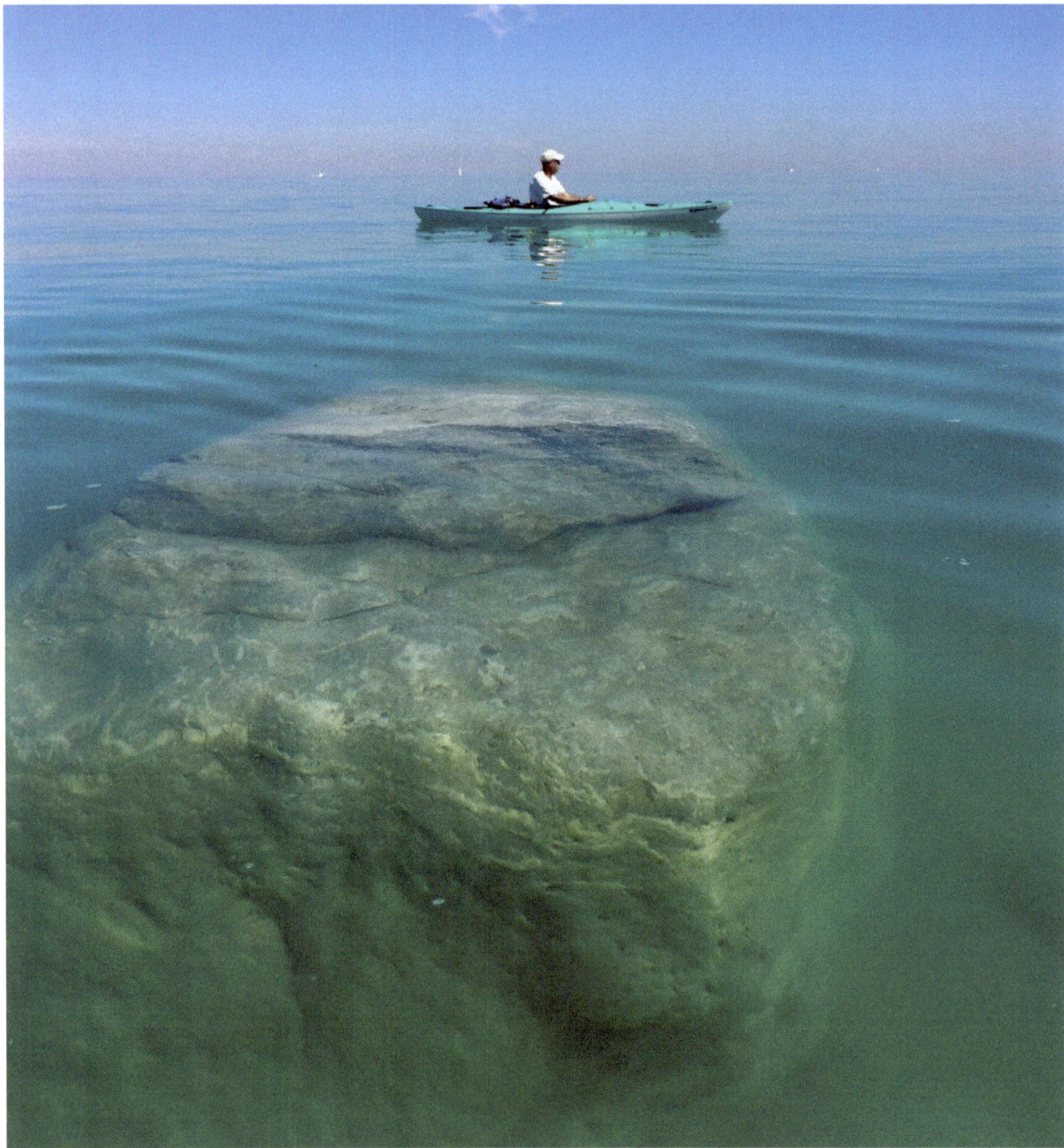

TRIP 7: GILLS PIER TO CATHEAD POINT

This trip began with our putting in at the dead end of Onomonee Road on a gorgeous July day when the water was calm as glass. Just offshore, there was a long spit of land that had been partially submerged by the rising levels of the Great Lakes. The image of the water, the narrow section of land near shore and the sky's horizon created a very interesting picture. This trip turned out to be one of our best adventures.

DATE OF TRIP: July 25, 2017

LOCATION: This section of day trips completes the western shoreline of the Leelanau peninsula, north of Leland.

ACCESS: The southern access point is the beach at the end of Onomonee Road. The best way to find the beach is to take M-22 north out of Leland (or south from Northport) and, at Fischer's Happy Hour Tavern, resist the temptation to turn in for some roasted chicken or a juicy hamburger. Instead, go north on Gills Pier Road. This road will dead-end at Onomonee Road (less than 2 miles). Turn left and you are right at the beach.

- The northern access point is at Christmas Cove Township Park. This beach and parking area is a bit more difficult to get to, but well worth your effort. Head north about a mile out of Northport on M-201 and turn left on Kilcherman Road. Kilcherman Road turns into Christmas Cove Road heading west. Continue about a mile to the parking area. There is plenty of parking, bathroom facilities and a beautiful sandy beach.

- Peterson Park is a popular place and a bit closer to Gills Pier. It could also be used as an access point. Be aware, though, that there is a much steeper and higher set of steps to negotiate in order to get to the water.

DISTANCE/TIME: Our trip from the Onomonee Road beach access to Cathead Point was about 5.5 miles. We then paddled back to our Christmas Cove destination — about 1.5 miles. The trip took us just under 3 hours with near perfect conditions.

STRATEGIES: This trip follows the strategies described in the other day trips on Lake Michigan. The less wind, the better, and be the most concerned about winds from the north, northwest and southwest. South or east winds would be preferred. You could go either direction using two vehicles to keep the winds and waves at your back.

FEATURES:

» Gills Pier, like most towns in this region, began as a lumber town. Today, all that remains are some old pilings from its pier and the nearby St. Wenceslaus Church. William Gill built a lumber mill on Lake Michigan after the Civil War, and a post office was opened in 1883. The first St. Wenceslaus church was built out of wood in 1890 to serve the many Bohemians who had emigrated to the area. At its peak, Gills Pier had 12 houses, a general store and a post office. The post office closed in 1908 and Gills Pier faded into history. In 1941, some of the local Bohemians built a new St. Wenceslaus Church out of brick. You can visit the church at 8500 East Kolarik Road.

» The landscape becomes less elevated as you approach Cathead Point to the north. The shoreline also becomes sandier the further north you paddle.

» Peterson Park sits about 350 feet (and 114 wooden steps) above Lake Michigan. It has 1,000 feet of rocky shoreline. This is a Petoskey stone hunter's dream location. Above the shore, there is a picnic area, a playground and a viewing platform overlooking Lake Michigan.

» Christmas Cove Park has over 200 feet of sandy beach frontage and picnic, parking and bathroom areas. The high lake levels have caused some concern for the long-term viability of the parking area that is currently on a low ridge, a few feet above the shore. One rumor about the origin of the Christmas Cove name was that a plane crashed near here on Christmas Day in the 1940s.

» Our paddle here was on one of the most perfect days to be out on Lake Michigan. The clarity of the water was unbelievable, and I think captured some of the magic in the pictures I took of the rocks below the surface of the water. The visibility above the water was excellent as well. We saw the reflections of islands, boats and wakes from far away, caused by a thermal inversion bending the line of sight from distances as far away as 60 miles. (This is known as a superior mirage: an area of warm air over a layer of colder air near the surface of even colder Lake Michigan distorts light rays, bending them over the visible horizon. Weird, but you can look it up.) As we rested right at the tip of Cathead Point, we were also able to see very clearly the cement factory in Charlevoix, about 20 miles across the water to the northeast, and some white buildings in Harbor Springs, another 15 miles beyond. It was definitely a moment to savor.

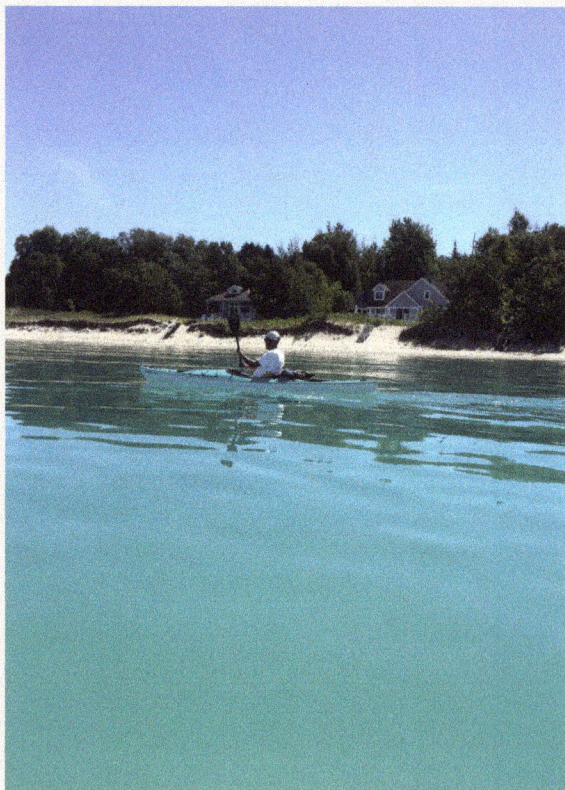

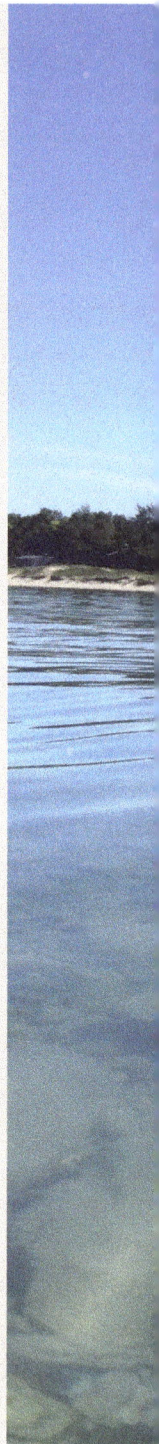

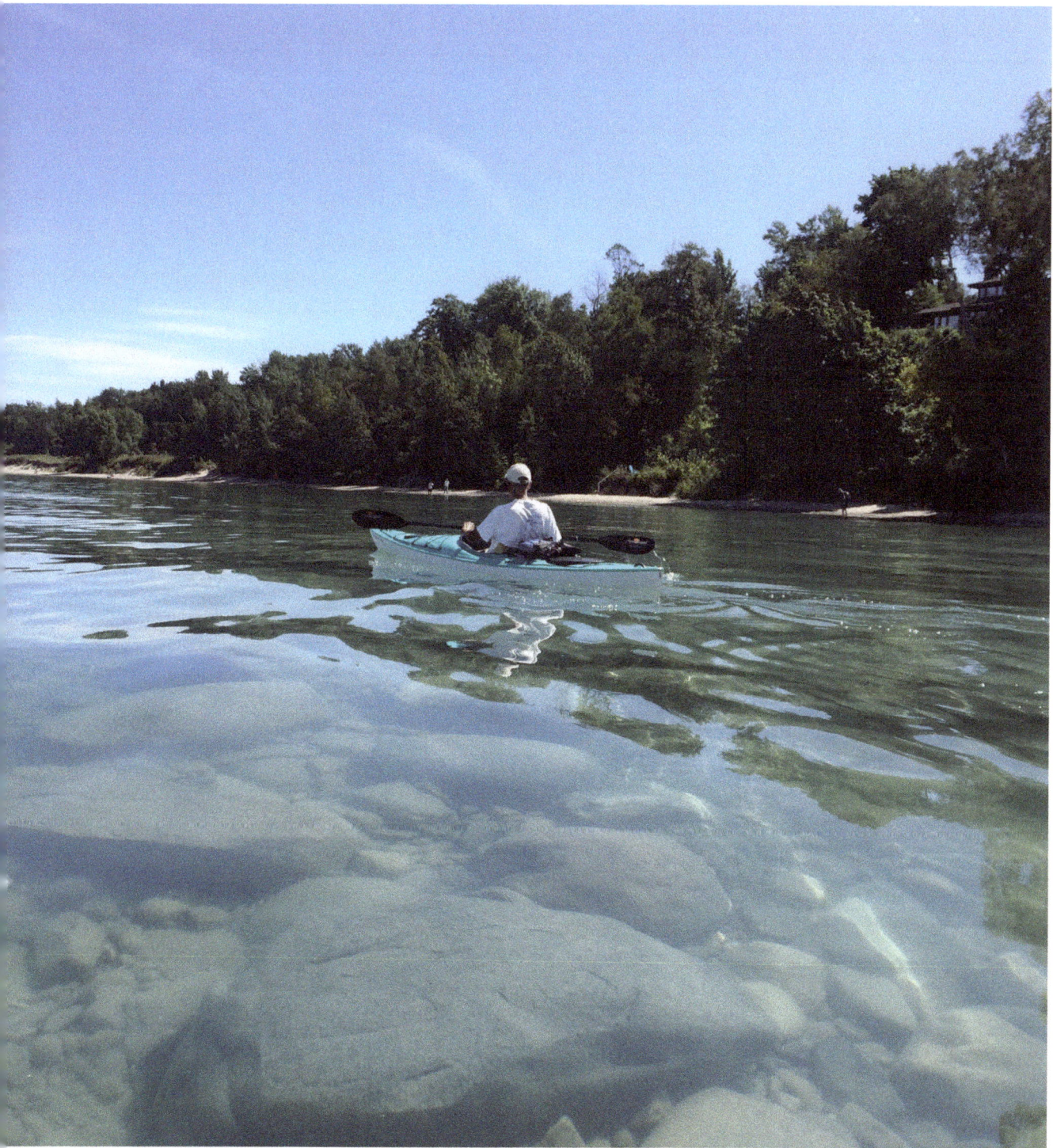

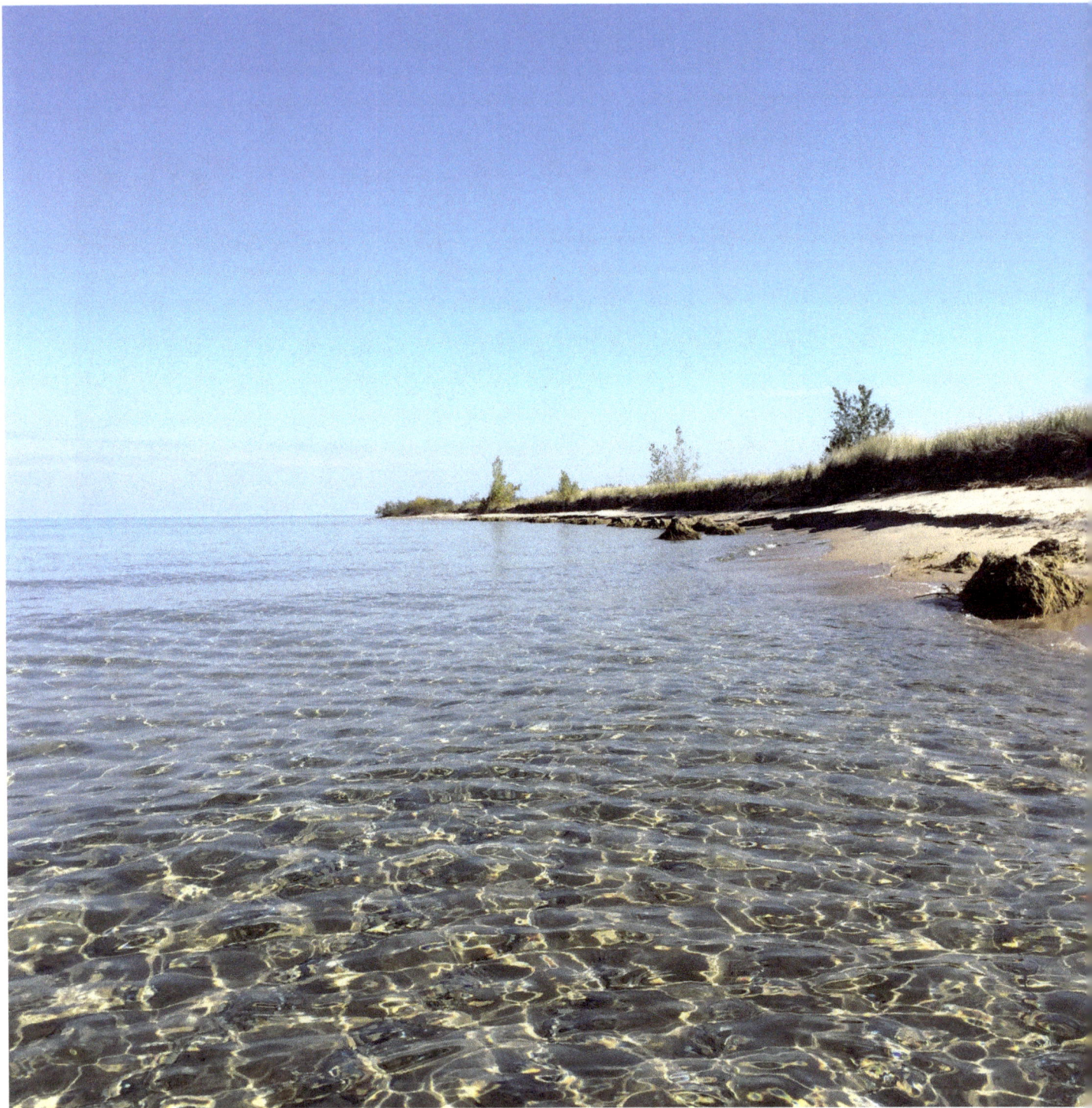

TRIP 8: THE TIP OF LEELANAU
TO CATHEAD POINT
GRAND TRAVERSE LIGHTHOUSE

This section was a very nice paddle along the low, sandy bluffs that are at the very northern tip of Leelanau County. There is much to see here, including many cottages and homes that sit just east of the Leelanau State Park. In the middle of these houses and cottages, there is a long stretch of state park land that is protected. This area probably looks as it was when the French explorers and fur traders paddled their canoes here in the 1700s — other than our kayaks, and maybe a nearby jet ski or sailboat.

DATE OF TRIP: September 25, 2015, September 5, 2019

LOCATION: This section is at the northern tip of Leelanau County. The Leelanau State Park and the Grand Traverse Lighthouse are 8.1 miles north of Northport.

ACCESS POINTS: The Leelanau State Park: this site requires a State Park sticker or a day pass. Both are available as you arrive. On our trip, we launched and returned to a rustic campsite. On another trip to this location, we used the beach closer to the lighthouse. We parked a vehicle in the main parking lot and carried our kayaks to a launch site.

- Christmas Cove Township Park (Described on Trip # 7): on this trip we met some kayakers who said that they had put in there, then paddled to the State Park Lighthouse.

STRATEGIES: Strong winds from the north, northwest, or northeast should be avoided. If we were to do this section again, I would use a two-vehicle strategy and either put in at Christmas Cove — if there was a west or southwest wind — and paddle to the State Park. With a southeast or east wind, I would put in at the Leelanau State Park and paddle west to Cathead Point and on towards Christmas Cove Township Park.

DISTANCE/TIME: Our paddle from Lighthouse Point to Cathead Point was approximately 5 miles and took us about 2 hours. The return trip was about the same in time.

- The distance from Cathead Point to the Christmas Cove Township Park is about 1.5 miles and would add another hour, depending on wind and wave conditions.

FEATURES:

» Cathead Bay's terrain is much different than the western shore of Leelanau. The dunes are lower and not as consistent and there are numerous sandy blowouts. The beach is narrow with some sand and rocks.

» The sand and gravel areas within the State Park land are marked as endangered piping plover nesting and feeding areas. These areas may be marked off as closed during the nesting months of May, June and July.

» If you're lucky enough to paddle here on a clear day, be sure to look for South Fox Island, 17 miles north of Cathead Point.

» The Grand Traverse Lighthouse was built in 1858, replacing an earlier round tower from 1852. Tours of the lighthouse and keeper's home are available, and there is a museum with exhibits on shipwrecks, the lighthouse and local history. The light can be seen from 8 miles away.

» The Leelanau State Park is a 1,740-acre recreation area at the northernmost extent of the Leelanau peninsula. The campground is rustic, with 51 campsites, 3 mini cabins and vault toilets. There are 8.1 miles of trails. The camping area is open from May 25 to November 4. In addition to the lighthouse and campground, there is a playground, a picnic area and a covered pavilion.

» One incident from this trip emphasizes my advice to always wear your life jacket on Lake Michigan. When we paddled here in the fall, we asked a park ranger at the entrance where we could launch our kayaks, and she said we could park in an empty campground site and follow one of the trails to Lake Michigan. Since the winds were very slight, I bungeed my life jacket behind the cockpit to drag the kayak through some rough underbrush to the shore. After launching, I noticed that I was taking on water. A repaired crack on the side of the kayak at the water line was leaking. Larry, being the more experienced kayaker, had a large sponge that I borrowed to bail out my kayak every 5 minutes or so. We continued across Cathead Bay to Cathead Point and back, repeating the process of stopping and bailing every 5 minutes. Back on the path through the woods to the car, Larry saw something on the ground, and said, "Hey, Jon, isn't that your life jacket?" Yes! I had paddled across some very deep water with a leaky boat, thinking the whole time that at least I had a life jacket right behind me if I needed it. The lessons are: 1) have something to bail out your kayak, and 2) always wear your life jacket on the Big Lake! You never know.

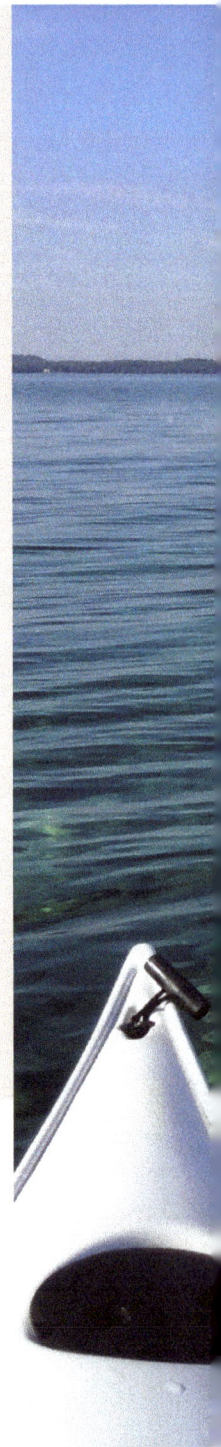

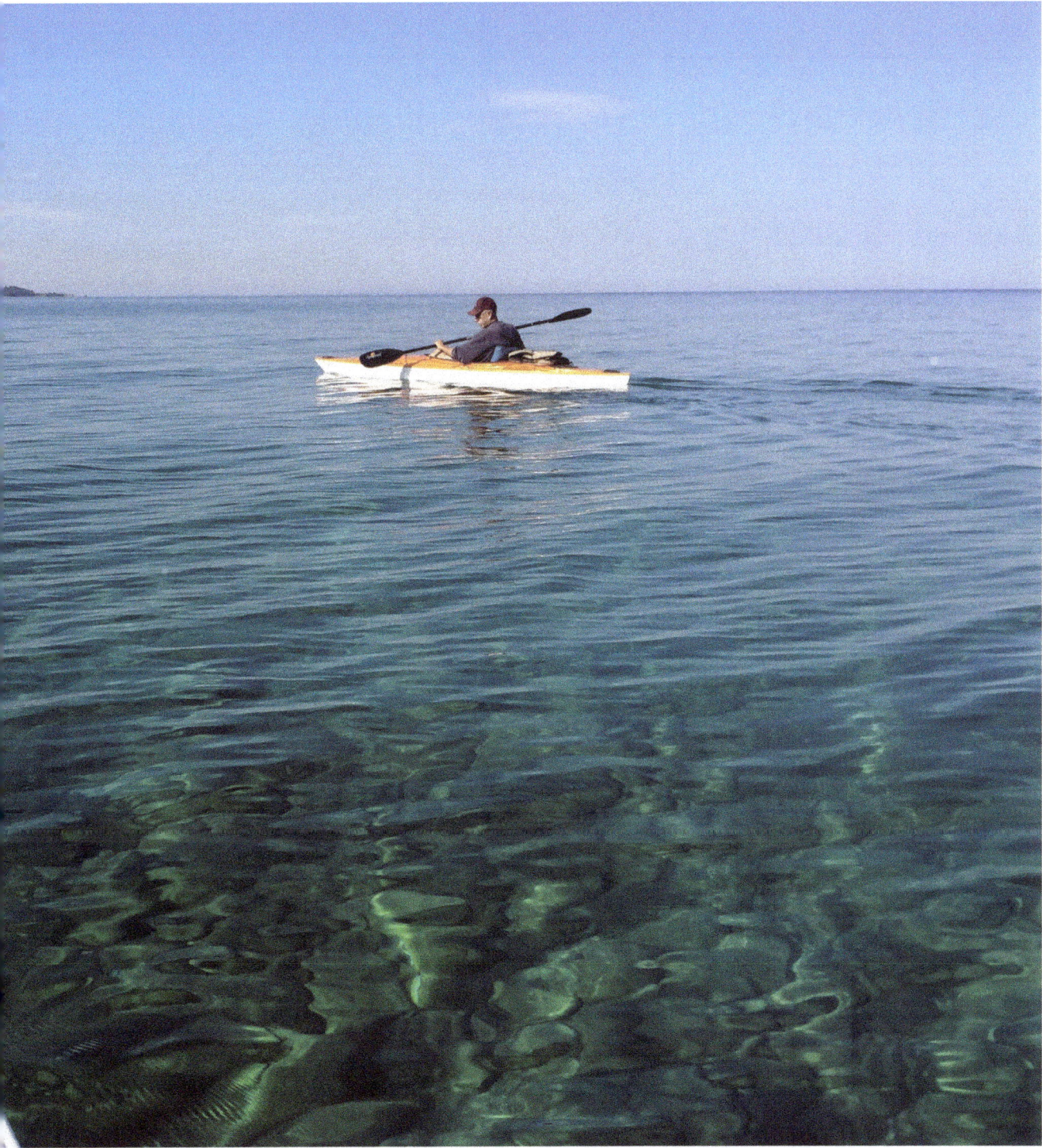

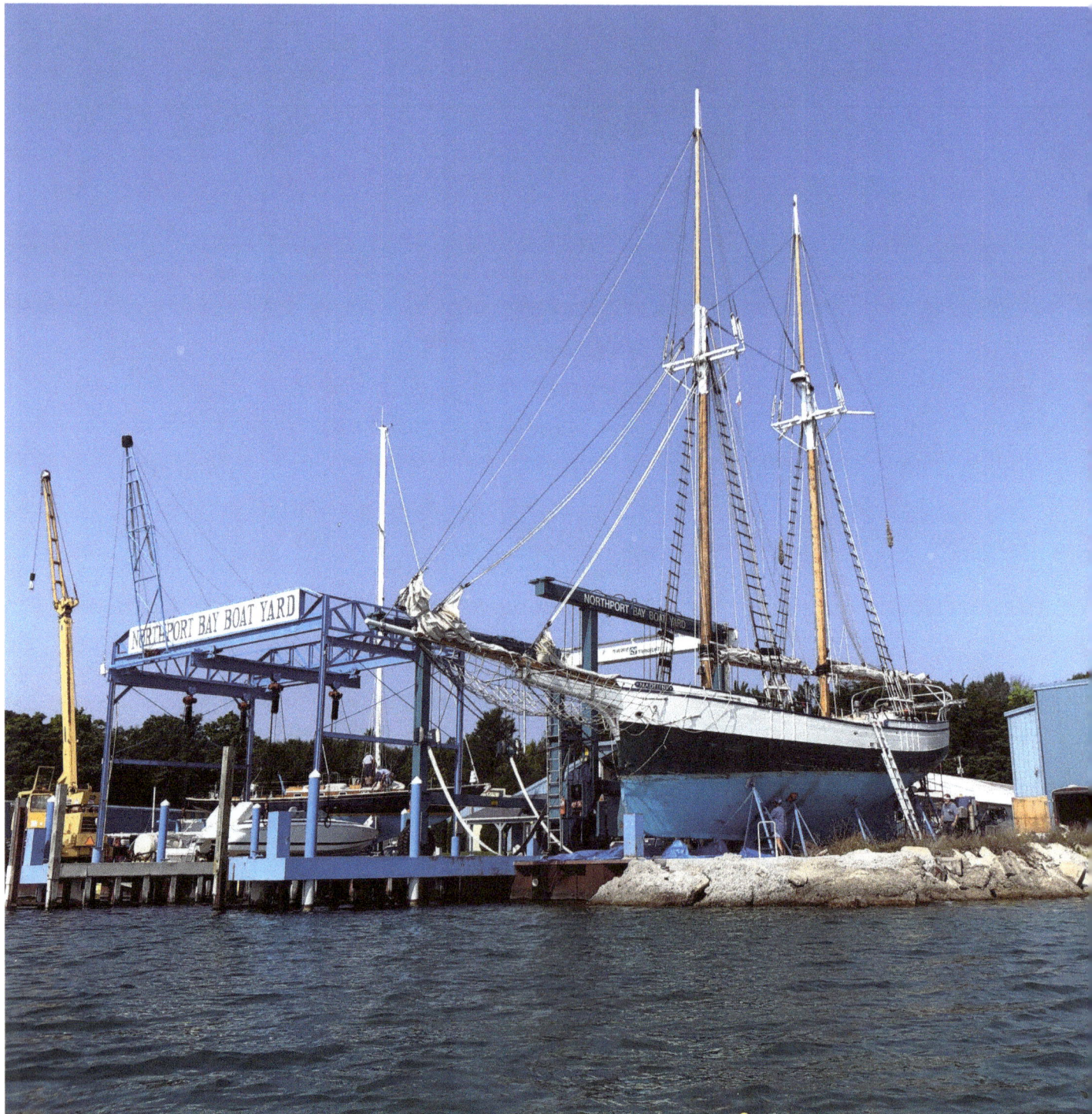

TRIP 9: NORTHPORT HARBOR TO THE LEELANAU LIGHTHOUSE

On this trip, we are venturing into the waters of Grand Traverse Bay. This bay got its name over 300 years ago from the French explorers and fur traders who, like Larry and me, tended to paddle close to shore. At 32 miles long and up to 10 miles wide, the French paddlers risked storms and dangerous waves to cross from what is now Antrim County to the tip of the Leelanau peninsula — the *grand traverse*. Our paddle from Northport to the Leelanau Lighthouse was about 14 miles, and we feel it is one of the most rewarding paddles in the area. The water of Grand Traverse Bay can be as pretty as the water of Lake Michigan, and the views go from the very rustic and remote to the landscaped wonders of large homes and estates. The amount of water traffic also goes from almost none, to some, to quite busy. The day we paddled there were lots of sailboats and power boats in the distance. And it was such a clear day that we could see the distant shores of Antrim county and the tip of The Old Mission Peninsula. This section is another wonderful way to explore Leelanau!

DATE OF TRIP: July 5, 2017

LOCATION: Northport is 26 miles north of Traverse City on M-22, 8.1 miles from the Leelanau State Park.

ACCESS POINTS: Northport has a sandy beach and park next to their marina, which is just east of the business district. There is plenty of parking and excellent restroom facilities.

- The access point at the other end of the trip is at the Leelanau State Park, described in detail in the previous day-trip.

DISTANCE AND TIME: The distance and time will vary depending on how you choose to get from Northport to Northport Point across Northport Bay. A direct line across is about 2 miles. If you choose to follow the shoreline, it's a little more than 4 miles. From Northport Point it's between 8 and 9 miles, following the shoreline to the lighthouse. We went almost directly across Northport Bay, and the trip took us 3.5 hours one-way.

STRATEGIES: Strategies are quite different on the Grand Traverse Bay side of Leelanau. Here, light winds from the southwest and northwest are the preferable conditions. With a two-vehicle strategy, the launch and landing sites can be switched — go from Northport to the lighthouse with a southern wind or go from the lighthouse to Northport with a northerly wind.

FEATURES:

» Some call the Grand Traverse Light at the Leelanau State Park the Cathead Light or the Northport Light. The original lighthouse was built in 1852. It was raided several times by Mormons from Beaver Island. In 1864 the lighthouse was torn down and replaced with the current one.

» A shoal extends north from Lighthouse Point several miles. In 1938, a 52-foot steel tower was built 2 miles northwest of the point. Its white light flashes every 6 seconds and can be seen from a distance of 7 miles.

» Northport is the first harbor at the northern end of Grand Traverse Bay. This harbor was a huge advantage in the early years, for boats seeking refuge and to purchase supplies of cordwood for their boilers. As we paddled, it was interesting to cross the shoal in the harbor and go from 80 feet deep to only 3 feet in just a few strokes! The colors of the water change dramatically with the changes of depth, and the rocks on the bottom are very beautiful to look at as you glide only a few feet above them. (There are several buoys to warn bigger boats of these shoals.)

» Northport was the first county seat of Leelanau County (from 1863 to 1883), and for a long time it was the largest community in the entire Grand Traverse region. The village was originally called Waukazooville, for the Native American Chief Waukazoo, who moved his people north from Holland because of a smallpox epidemic. The name was changed in 1854. The first cherries in the region were planted in the 1850s.

» This paddle also goes across the 45th Parallel. The line is just north of Northport at the narrowest section of Northport Point.

» Grand Traverse Bay's northern boundary is a line from Lighthouse Point to the Antrim-Charlevoix county line. The total water area of Grand Traverse Bay is 278.1 square miles. Its shoreline is 131 miles and the distance from Lighthouse Point to Clinch Park in Traverse City is 31 miles.

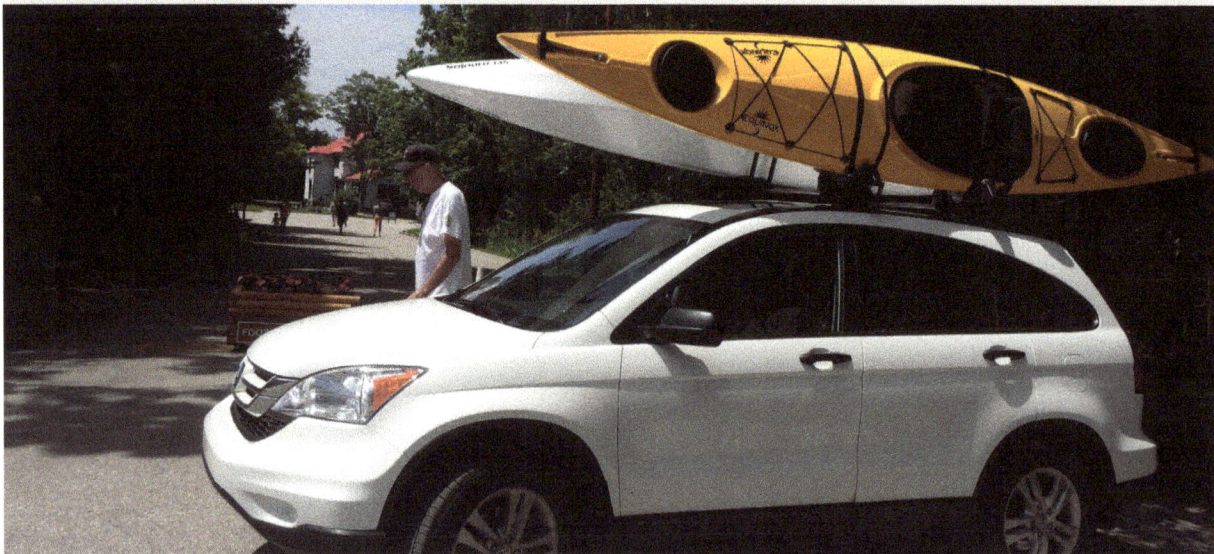

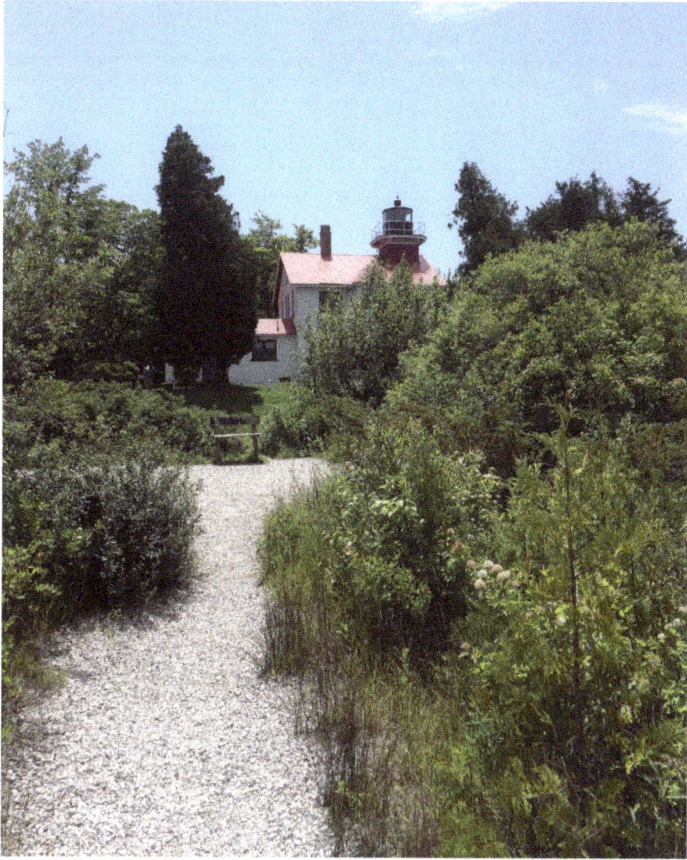

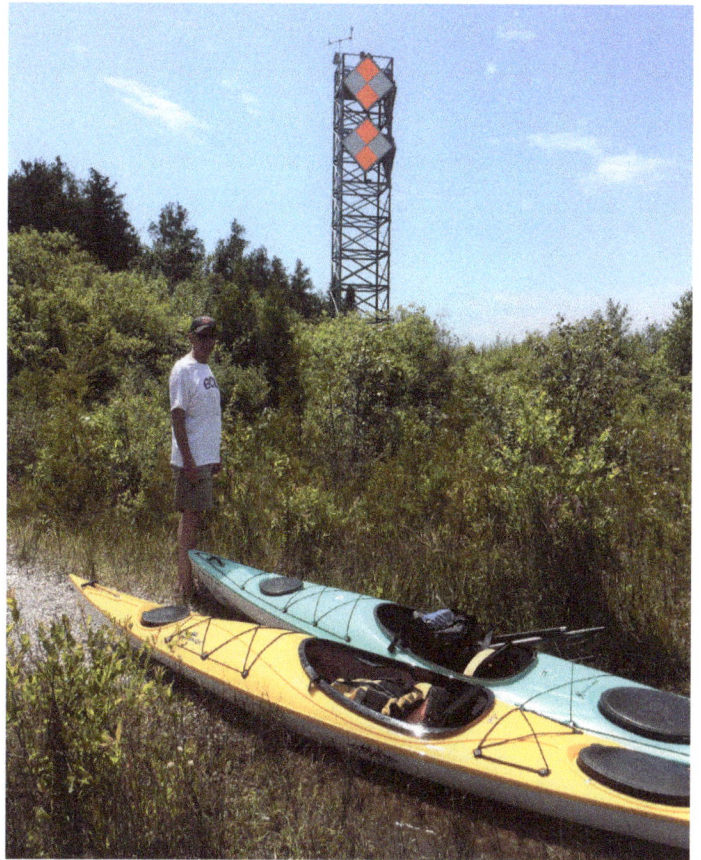

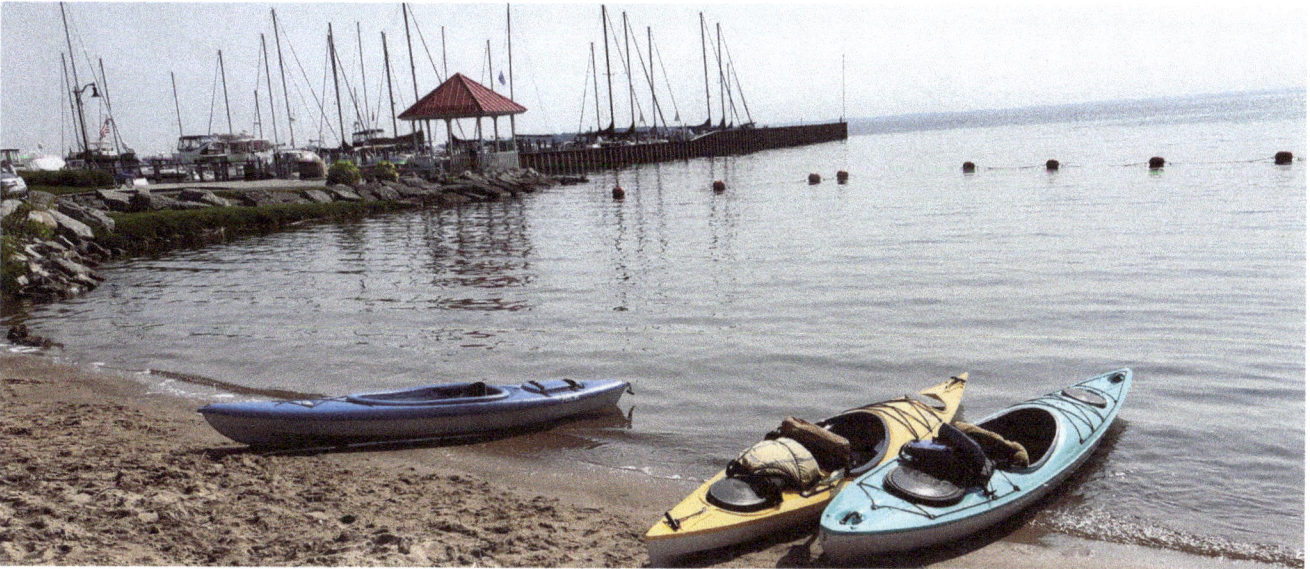

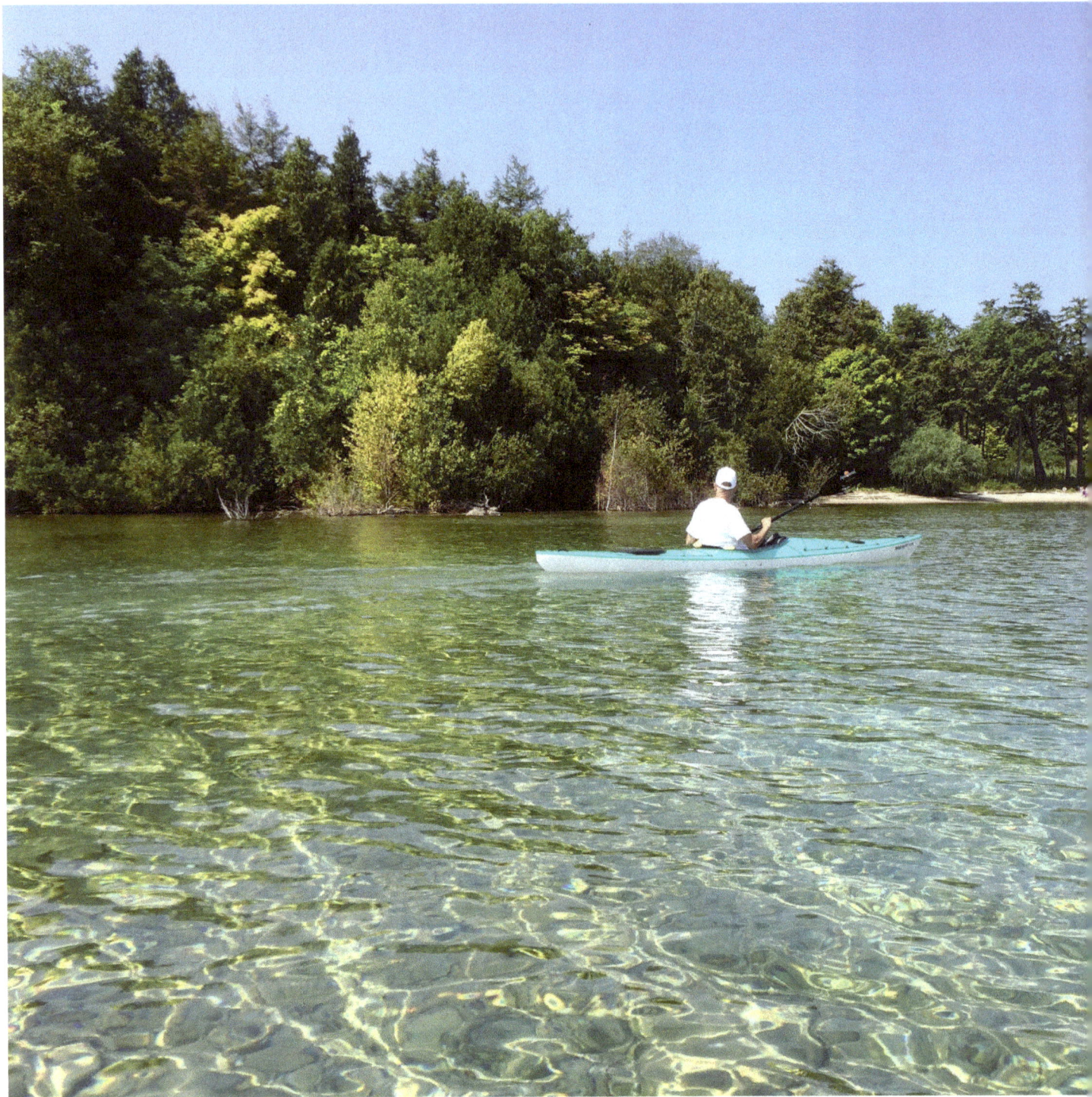

TRIP 10: OMENA TO NORTHPORT

This was one of our last paddles on the tour around Leelanau, and it was one of the finest. When you're traveling by car along M-22 between Omena and Northport, you don't get to see much of the water or shore. Paddling between the two gives you that view, and it is a very interesting one.

DATE OF TRIP: August 8, 2017

LOCATION: Omena is located 23 miles north of Traverse City on the New Mission Bay of Grand Traverse Bay. Northport is 26 miles north of Traverse City on Northport Bay.

ACCESS: Southern access point: There's a small township park and beach in Omena that's a great spot to launch a kayak. Located on Omena Point Road, east of M-22, it's in the business district of Omena. Parking is across the road from the beach. Portable toilets are available by the parking area.

- Northern access point: The best spot for launching a kayak in Northport is the Public Beach just east of the Central Business District and next to the Northport Marina. Drinking water and indoor toilets are available.

DISTANCE/TIME: This section is approximately 7.5 miles long, following the shoreline. It took us 3.5 hours in conditions of slightly increasing winds from the west as we rounded the northern part of Omena Point.

STRATEGIES: This section is well protected from winds from the southwest, west, and northwest.

- With a two-vehicle strategy, the direction of the trip could be changed depending on a north or south wind.
- There are many fine places to get food and refreshments near either access point.

FEATURES:

» Omena was founded in 1852 when the Reverend Peter Daugherty relocated his Indian Mission from Old Mission, on the tip of Old Mission Peninsula. New Mission was the name he chose for his new location across Grand Traverse Bay. A post office was established in 1858. The name was later changed to Omena — an Ojibwe expression for "Is that so?" and supposedly Reverend Daugherty's favorite expression in response to comments by his parishioners. The Presbyterian Church still is there and continues Sunday services.

» Omena has historical ties to two Civil War generals: Major General George A. Custer and Brigadier General Benjamin H. Grierson. Custer's connection to Omena is due to his marriage to Elizabeth Clift Bacon of Monroe, Michigan, whose family were among the first to own land in Omena and Omena Point in the 1850s. General Custer likely only visited Omena once, in July of 1864, to visit relatives. General Benjamin Grierson's 6th Illinois Cavalry's most famous Civil War action was in Mississippi, in April of 1863, during Grant's siege of Vicksburg. Known as "Grierson's Raid," he led 1,700 men and destroyed Confederate supplies and infrastructure. Grant called his action "one of the most brilliant cavalry exploits of the war." In 1890, Grierson retired from the military and, in 1896, he built a summer cottage that he called "The Garrison." Around 1890, he bought land on the Point and operated the cottage as a hotel called "The Oaks." Grierson died in Omena on August 31, 1911.

» Across from New Mission Bay is the Omena Traverse Yacht Club. This is a center of social life in the area.

» Ahgosatown Landing is a Marina and RV Park between Omena and Northport at 6490 N. West Bay Shore Drive.

» Bellow (or Gull or Trout or Fisher's) Island is located about 1.5 miles off the Leelanau Peninsula shore and about 3 miles south of Northport. It's a mysterious-looking island with an abandoned house and two tall chimneys, all visible from your kayak. The house was built around 1910, by Edward Ustick, Sr., from St. Louis, Missouri. Despite warnings about the seagulls, he was quoted as saying, "the gulls would have to go." The house was designed by Traverse City architect Jens C. Petersen, and materials were hauled over the frozen bay by horse-drawn sledges — while the gulls were absent. The two fieldstone chimneys were constructed by Byron Woolsey, who also did work at Northport Point's Atwill Memorial Chapel and the Woolsey Memorial Airport. The Ustick family summered off and on at the island retreat, but stopped visiting the island around the time of WWII. In August of 1948, vandals entered and wrecked the cottage with axes. Six juveniles from the resort colony at Northport Point admitted to the act. For many years the property sat vacant, passing through different owners. Meanwhile, the gulls had no competition for their rookery. No doubt the 1963 Hitchcock movie, "The Birds," had an impact on the reluctance of others to rebuild on the island. In 1995, the Leelanau Land Conservancy acquired the island.

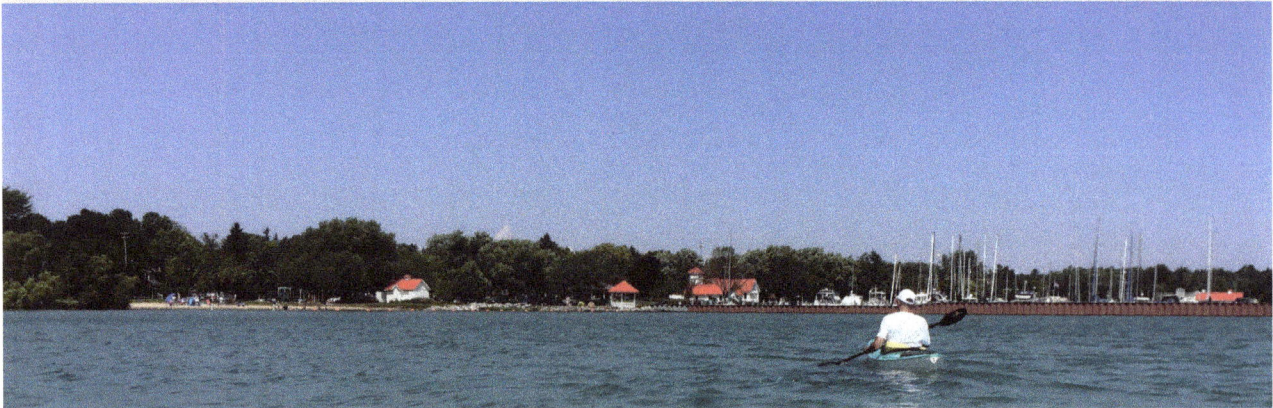

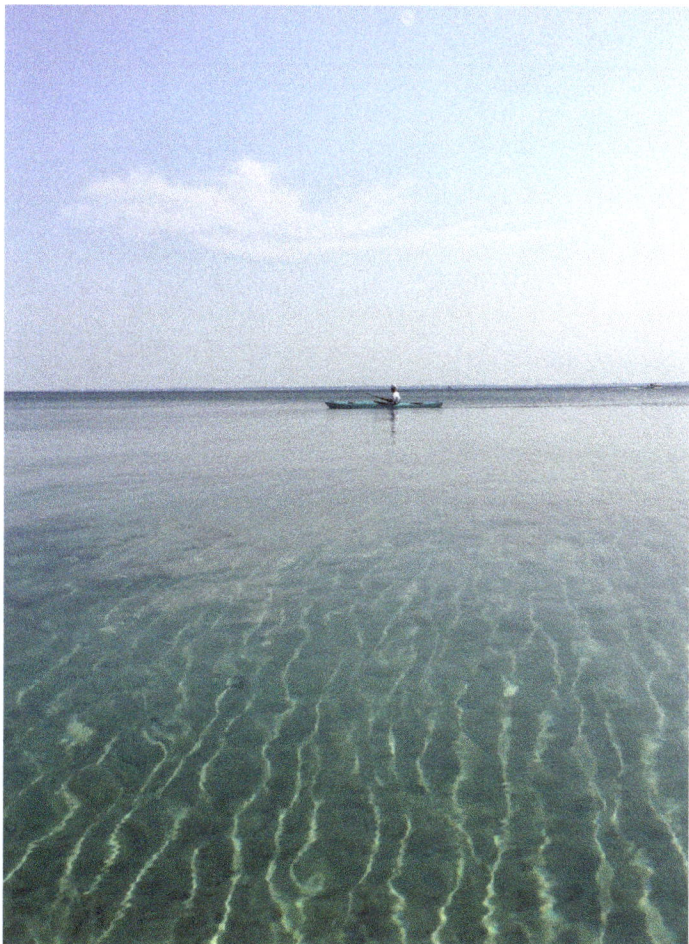

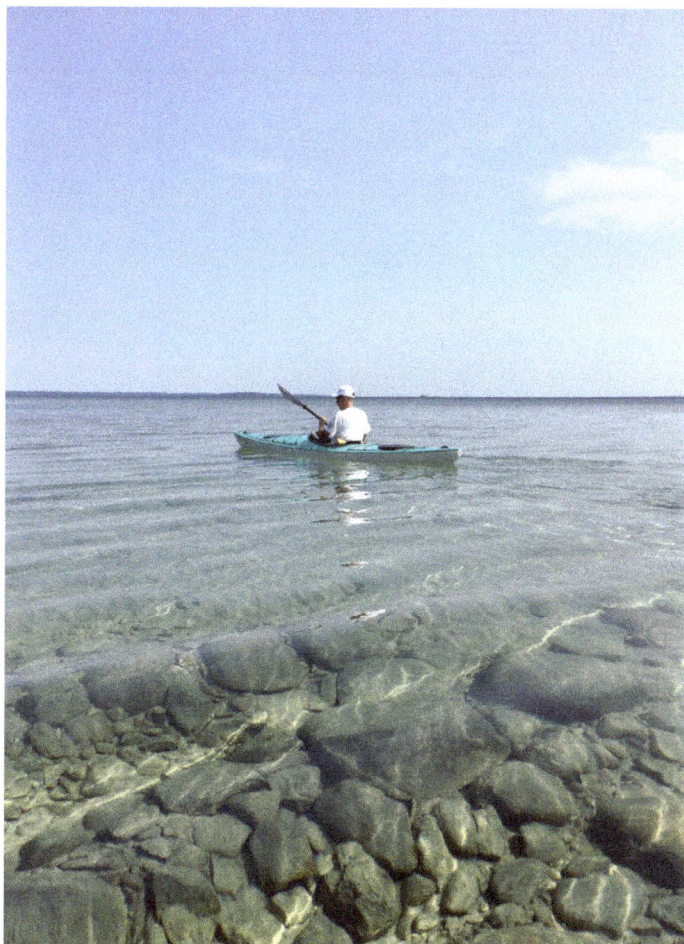

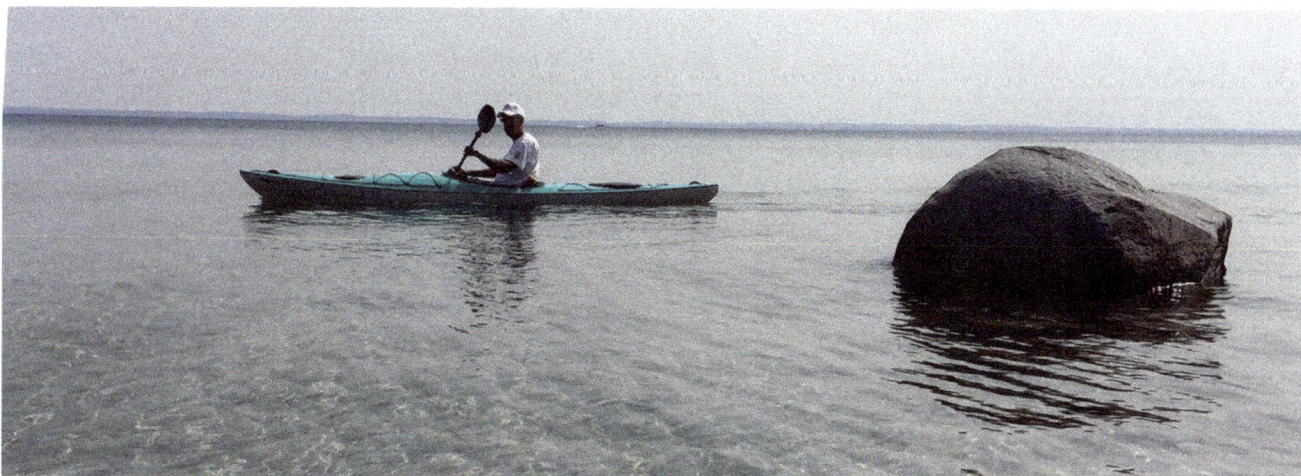

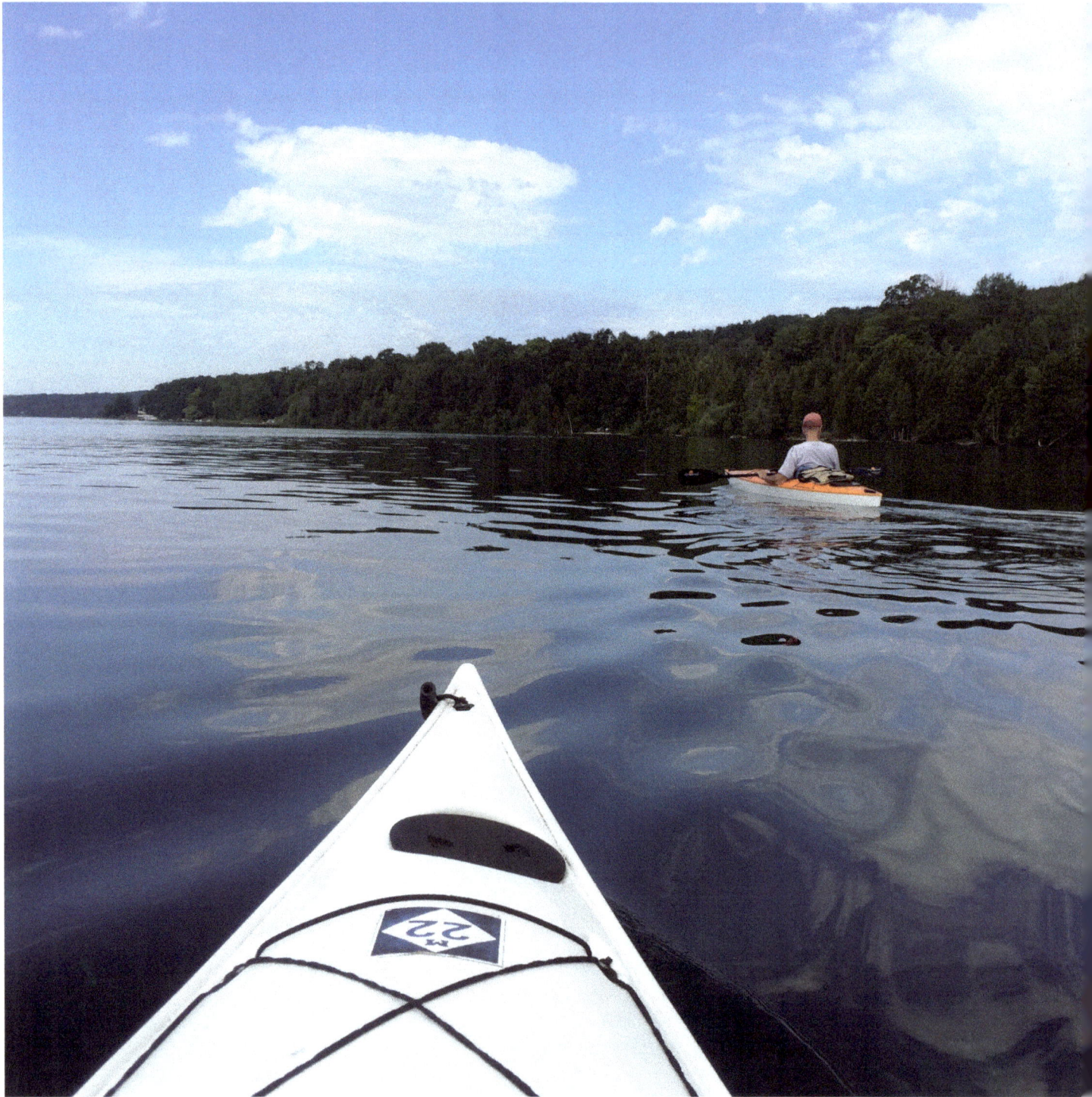

TRIP 11: OMENA TO SUTTONS BAY

This is a great spot to visit, especially when the westerly winds are too high for other areas. Omena Bay and Suttons Bay are both famous for their beautiful, clear, pristine water. On the day we paddled, there was an almost laser-like streaking in the water created by a combination of reflecting ripples from our paddles and the wake off the bow of the lead kayak.

DATE OF TRIP: July 27, 2016

LOCATION: Suttons Bay is 17 miles north of Traverse City on M-22. It is one of the protected harbors on West Grand Traverse Bay.

ACCESS: The northern access point is the small township park in Omena, just off M-22 on Omena Point Road.

- The southern access point is Sutton Park, also known as South Shore Park in Suttons Bay. The park has 300 feet of shoreline, as well as public bathrooms, a playground and a picnic shelter.

- Other options include 45th Parallel Park, north of the village of Suttons Bay. This is a tiny picnic area with limited parking.

- Village Marina Park Complex in Suttons Bay is at the end of Adams Street. There's parking, a sandy beach, a bathhouse and restrooms.

- Graham Green Park is located 3 miles north of Suttons Bay along M-22. The beach is mostly rocky, with occasional sandy sections. There is parking, plus picnic tables and grills. Porta Potties are provided.

DISTANCE/TIME: The shoreline distance is approximately 8 miles. It took us about 2.15 hours to go from Omena to Suttons Bay in calm winds and flat water.

STRATEGIES: The nice thing about Suttons Bay is that it is well-protected from all directions except the east. If there are more northerly winds, put in at Omena and go south. If winds are more southerly, do the opposite. This paddle is a great alternative when there are stronger winds from any westerly direction.

FEATURES:

» Suttons Bay has had three names. In 1867, it was originally called Suttonsburg. In 1871, It was named Pleasant City and there were plans to locate a national university on the bay. In the 1870s the town was renamed Suttons Bay.

» The waters of Omena Bay are an uncommon, deep purple in deep areas.

» The tip of Old Mission Peninsula comes more in focus the closer you get to Suttons Bay.

» Peshawbestown is a community known today as the home of the Leelanau Sands Casino. It began as a Catholic mission to the people of the Chippewa and Ottawa tribes around 1850. Its first name was Eagletown, then changed to Peshawbestown to honor the ruling chief Peshaba. The casino and Native American museum can be seen from the water. There is a private marina just north of Peshawbestown.

» The village of Suttons Bay has a population of 608, and is a favorite tourist destination. This village was named after Harry C. Sutton, a lumberman who came to the area in 1854. Today, Suttons Bay has a movie theater, many shops and restaurants. Bahles is a local clothing store that has been a family operation since 1876.

» Just north of Suttons Bay there is a road sign marking the 45th parallel north. Here you are halfway between the Equator and the North Pole.

» We paddled this section in 90-degree heat and lots of humidity. A good reminder is to use sunblock and always bring sunglasses and a good hat. We took a few rest breaks to drink some water and enjoy the views.

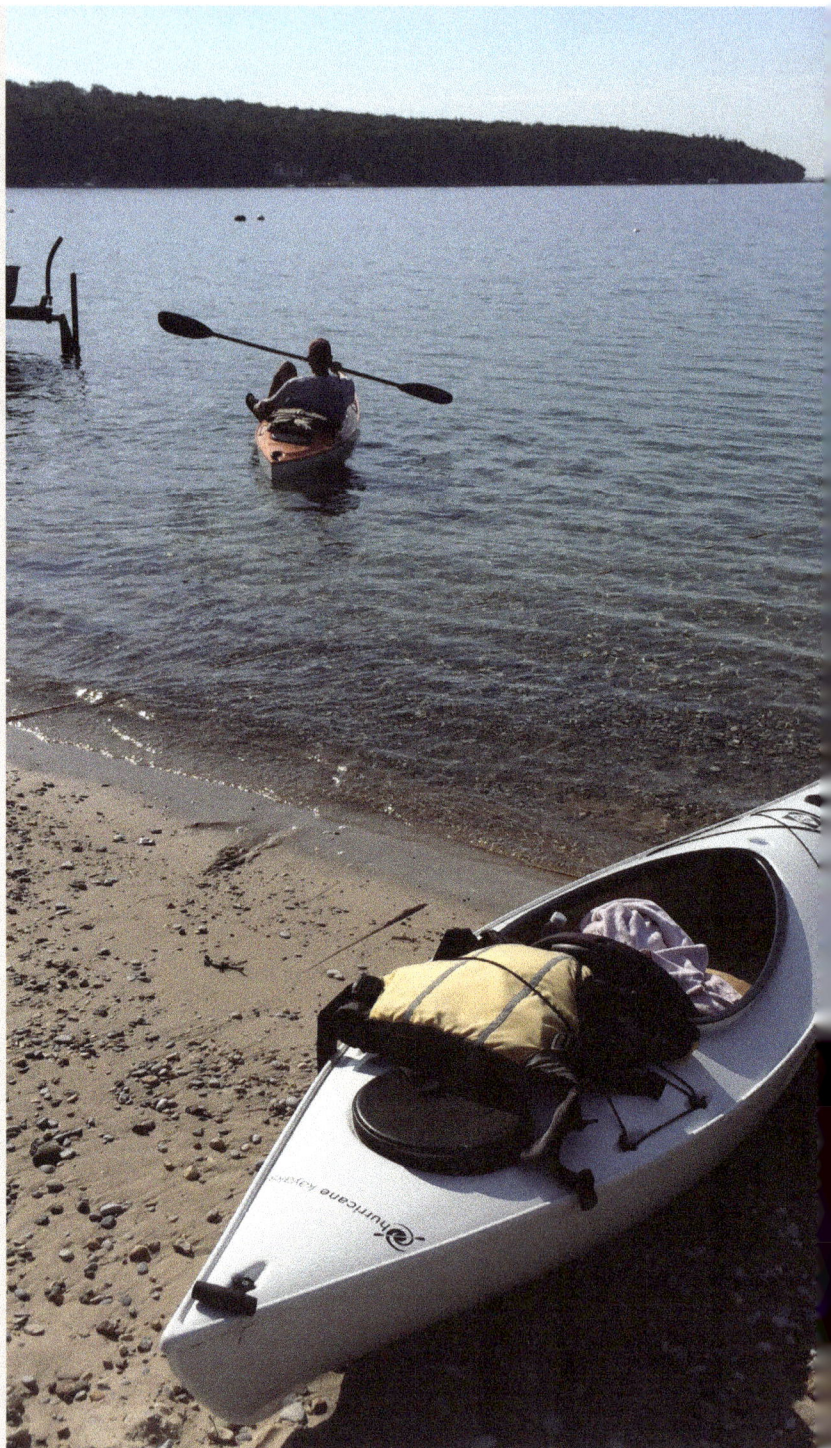

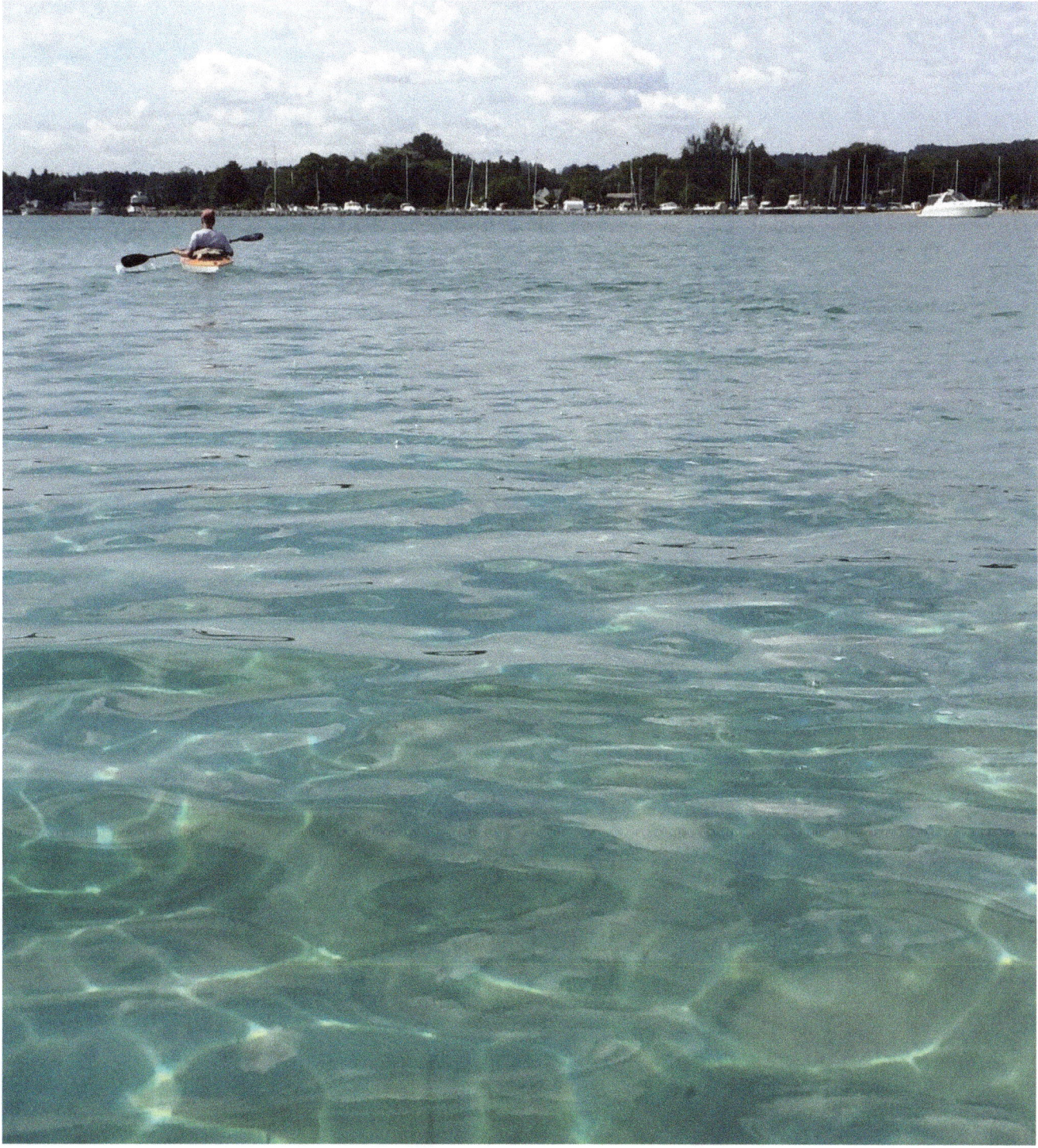

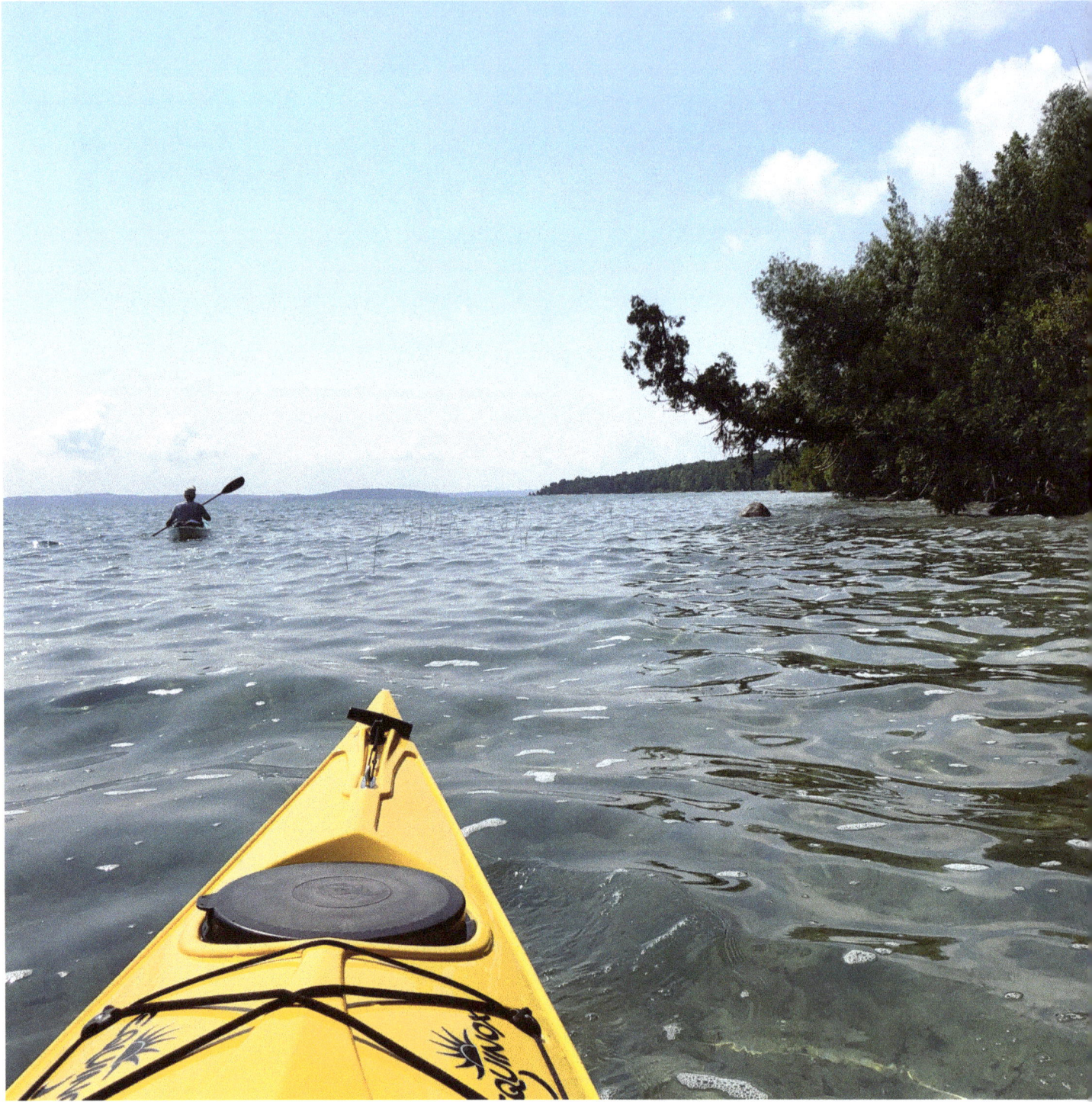

TRIP 12: LEE POINT TO SUTTONS BAY

This section includes the protected waters in Suttons Bay and the more open waters of West Grand Traverse Bay. There are many boats and other watercraft to see, especially closer to Suttons Bay. The tree-covered bluffs that face Grand Traverse Bay feature many fine homes. The water is extremely clear, and there are many rocks and boulders to be seen below the surface. From Lee Point, the more urban skyline of Traverse City comes into view to the south.

DATE OF TRIPS: June 16, 2014; September 8, 2014 (with Dave Clinton)

LOCATION: Lee Point is about 11 miles from Traverse City.

ACCESS: There are several access locations on this section. They include:

- Sutton Park, just south of the business district of Suttons Bay at M-22 and Park Street.
- Lover's Lane Park is a small sliver of property that gives access to the waters of Suttons Bay. It is located off of Stoney Point Road, near the tip of Stoney Point — the peninsula that juts into the bay. There is limited parking and there are no amenities.
- Vic Steimel Park is a one-acre park also located at the tip of Stoney Point. There is a small landing, a picnic area with tables and grills and Porta Potties.
- Hendryx Park is an excellent place to launch a kayak. Located just east of M-22 and Lee Point Road, the park has picnic tables and grills.
- There is a DNR boat launch at the junction of Hilltop Road and M-22 with parking and restrooms.
- Boughey Park, at the eastern end of Bingham Road and M-22, is another option. There's a playground, a covered pavilion and Porta Potties.

DISTANCE AND TIMES:

- Our first trip was from Hendryx Park to Lover's Lane Park and return — a round trip distance of approximately 10 miles. It took us about 3 hours.
- The second trip started at Vic Steimel Park. We paddled past the business district, then directly across the bay and back to the launch site. Round trip was approximately 6 miles and took less than 2 hours.

STRATEGIES: A two-vehicle strategy could be used by spotting a vehicle at Hendryx or Vic Steimel Park, then launching from one of the access sites near or north of Suttons Bay. (Or vice versa, depending on the wind.)

FEATURES:

» If you draw a straight line from Suttons Point (Stony Point) to Old Mission Point, then continue that to Antrim County, you get what would be an arbitrary line defining the East and West Bays in Grand Traverse Bay. By using this line for a northern marker, West Bay measures 61.2 square miles and East Bay 60.9 square miles. The rest of Grand Traverse Bay — north of that line to the line from Lighthouse Point to Antrim County — is 156 square miles. (Mapping Unlimited data)

» The Old Mission Peninsula and Power Island to the east are easily viewed on this trip. They are about 3 to 4 miles away, and the paddle takes you parallel to them.

» Like much of Leelanau County, this is a prime fruit-growing area. Cherries, apples and grapes are harvested here. Leelanau is also wine country. Hops are increasingly grown.

» This eastern stretch of the Leelanau Peninsula shore is one of the quietest. North and south of this paddle, M-22 and its traffic hug the shoreline. You kind of get used to the constant rumbling of cement trucks, buses, cars and R-Vs, but it's also great to get to places where all you hear are the sounds of the paddle splashing the water, waves on the shore and seagulls calling out from above.

» The day Dave Clinton and I paddled together, we shared the bay with the tall ship schooner, *The Inland Seas*, which docks in Suttons Bay. This is a teaching and research vessel operated by the Inland Seas Education Association, a non-profit organization dedicated to helping people of all ages experience the Great Lakes.

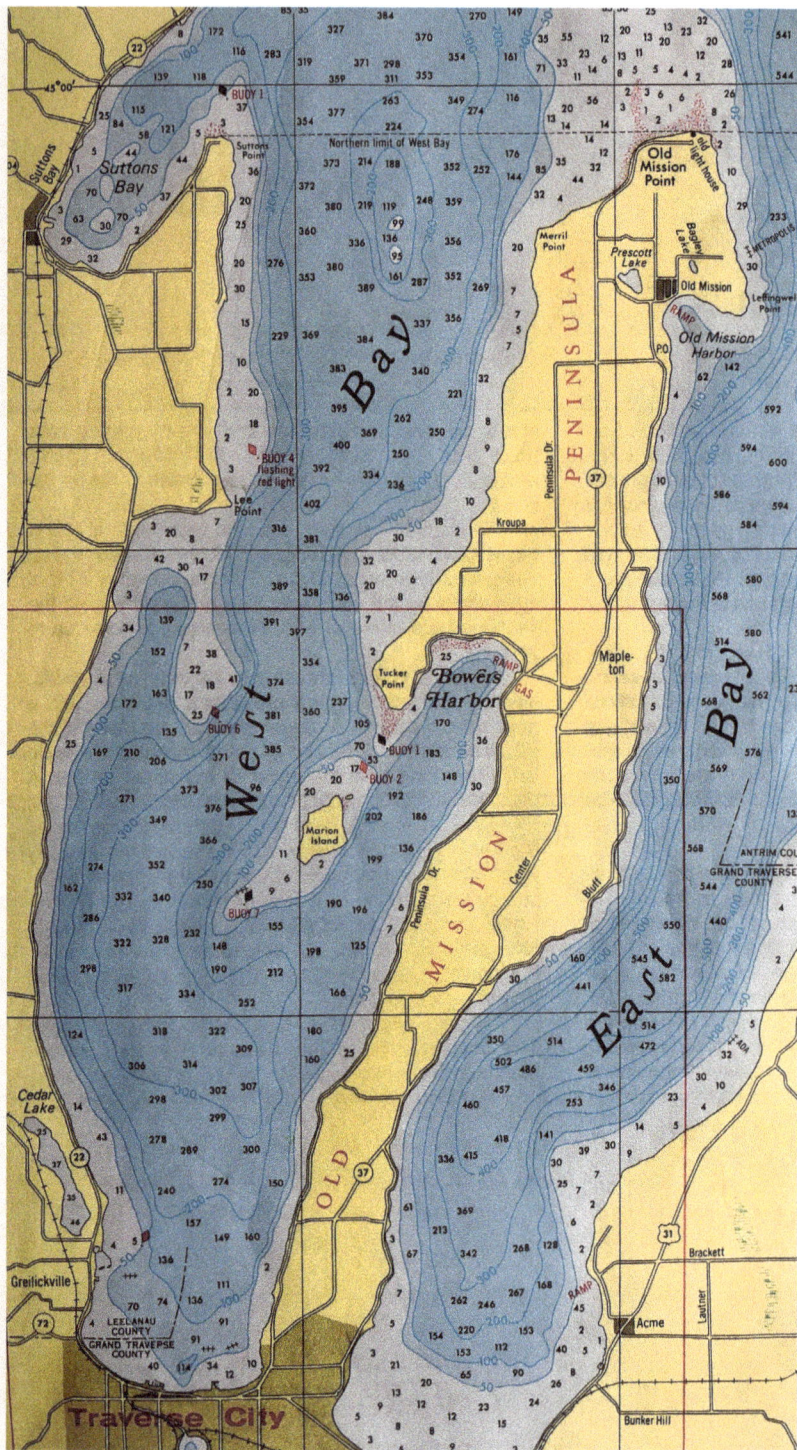

TRIP 13: LEE POINT
TO PATHFINDER SCHOOL

This is one of the last legs on our tour of the shoreline of Leelanau. Here, the paddling follows parallel to M-22 as the highway hugs the eastern shoreline. As we traveled just off-shore from this busy road, I wondered if some of the drivers and passengers in the vehicles thought about how nice it would be to trade places with us out on the bay. M-22 is a great drive, and I have been on that road many times, but I know I prefer to be the one in the kayak, on the water, looking at the shoreline — especially with the great conditions we had on the day we paddled there.

DATE OF TRIP: July 11, 2017

LOCATION: This section runs from near Cherry Bend Road (about 2 miles north of Traverse City) to Cherry Cove on West Bay (about 11 miles from Traverse City).

ACCESS: There are several options is this section of where to put in and take out.

- Hendryx Park on Lee Point Road, one mile east of M-22.

- Boughey Park on M-22, at the end of Bingham Road. This park has 50 feet of frontage and can be used to launch a kayak. There is parking, as well as picnic facilities and a pit toilet.

- There are two roadside picnic sites with access to West Bay. One is 2.1 miles north of the stop light at the M-22 and M-72 intersection in Traverse City. The other is 4.0 miles north of there. Both have limited parking and steps to the beach. There are no bathroom facilities.

TIME AND DISTANCE: Paddling from the Hendryx Park to the access point across from Pathfinder School is about 9 miles. We've also paddled from Boughey Park to the Pathfinder School access point and it was about 8 miles. The latter took us about 2.75 hours in hot but very calm conditions.

STRATEGIES: This is one of the most protected areas from most prevailing winds. The bluffs are fairly high, limiting the problems caused by westerly winds. With a two-car strategy, you could choose to travel in either direction if there is an issue with northeast or southerly winds.

» The homes and estates on the shore and on the bluffs overlooking the bay are very nice. Many of the homes are separated by M-22 from the water but have water access.

» Just a few years ago, the water level of Lake Michigan — and hence Grand Traverse Bay — was very low. In fact, in January, 2013, it was at an historical, all-time low. Since then, levels have rebounded nearly 4 feet, partially because of increased ice cover in winter and above average precipitation. (Levels are currently still 2 feet below the record set in 1986.) Periods of extremes — whether high or low — cause problems. Too low, and there are issues of boat access to harbors and hoists. Also, the exposed shoreline increases the amount of problem vegetation. Too high, and there is the potential for erosion and property damage or loss. The good news is that changing water levels have little effect on kayaking. "Paddle on" in whatever current lake level exists.

» Pathfinder School is an independent, alternative school (pre-kindergarten through 8th grade), established in 1972. It is located on M-22, directly across from the access point we used on our paddle.

» Greilickville, just north of Traverse City, is an unincorporated community with a population of 1,415. It was first called "Norristown," after Seth and Albert Norris who built a gristmill here in 1853. Then Godfrey Greilick and his sons built a sawmill in the mid-1850s, and the name changed. The mill became one of the most important in the region, cutting 8.5 million feet of hardwood in 1883. Soon, Greilickville also had a brickyard, a brewery, a tannery, a hospital and a railroad station on the Manistee and Northeastern Railroad line.

» Larry and I have both noticed an increase in the clarity of the water on our recent day trips. An October 6, 2017, article in the *Detroit News* reported that Lake Michigan and Lake Huron have both surpassed Lake Superior in water clarity. It stated that this was the result of climate changes, less phosphorus runoff and an increase in zebra and quagga mussel filtration of plankton.

» One of the highlights for me on this trip was paddling past a home that was on my list of possible homes to purchase back in the mid-1970s. It was interesting to consider how things could have been different had I chosen to live on Grand Traverse Bay rather than Cedar Lake.

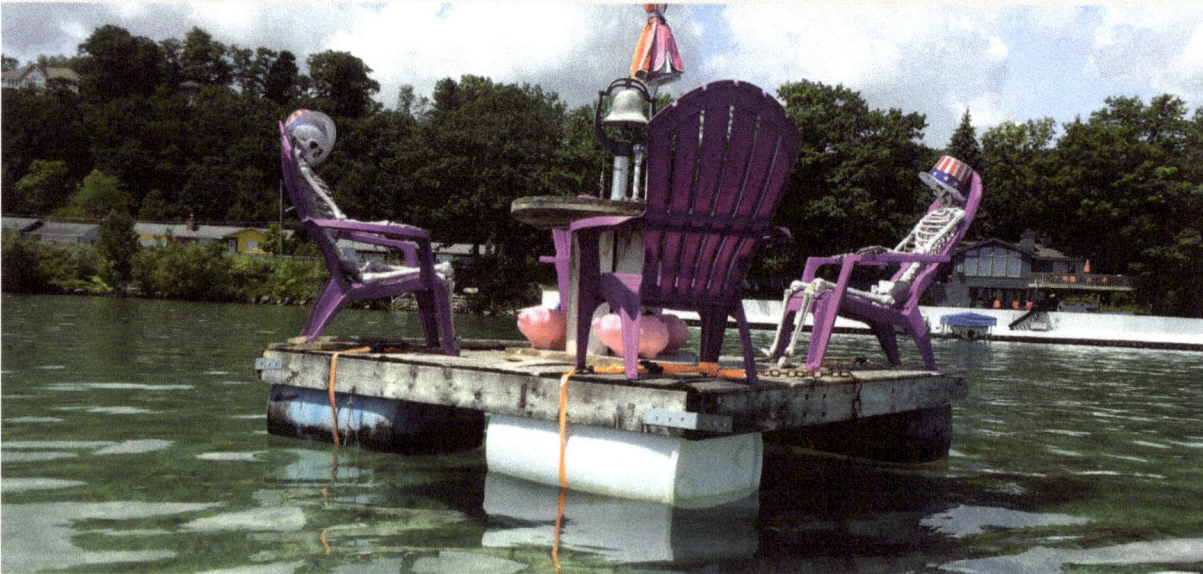

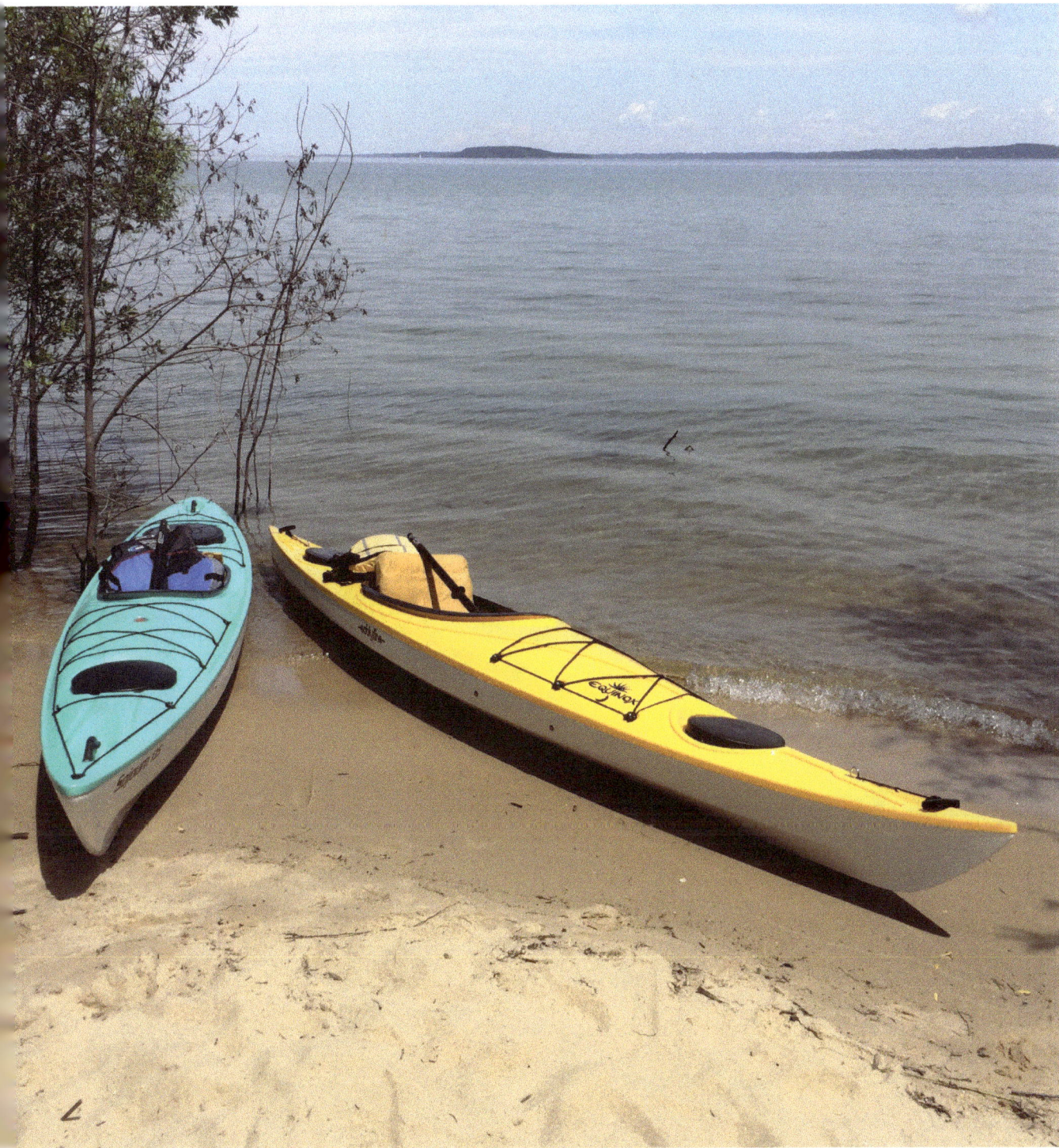

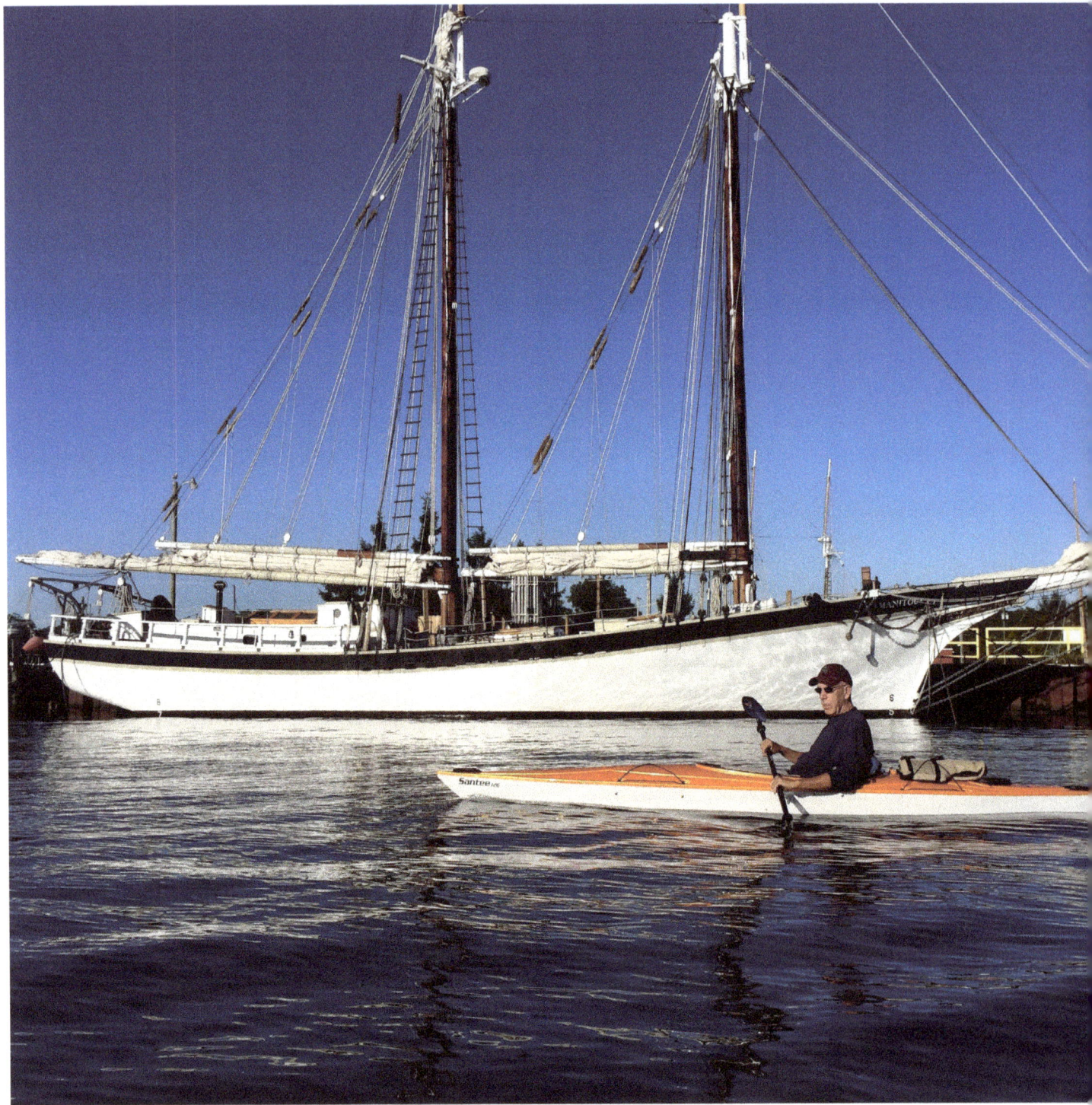

TRIP 14: GREILICKVILLE TO CLINCH PARK
TRAVERSE CITY

This trip is the most urban of them all. It includes some of the tallest buildings in northern Michigan —which definitely gives the paddle a different vibe. Still, the water is pure and the scenery is wonderful. It's great looking across the bay at the Old Mission Peninsula, or north to Power Island, or just taking in the skyline and the beaches of Traverse City.

DATE OF TRIP: September 30, 2016

LOCATION: This is the closest trip from Traverse City — right on its northern doorstep.

ACCESS: There are several options in choosing where to start and end this section:

- North of Traverse City, there are the several sites mentioned in the day-trip from Lee Point to Pathfinder that one could use for access to West Grand Traverse Bay.

- The site we used was Elmwood Township Park, located next to the Elmwood Township Marina, about 0.9 miles north of Traverse City on M-22. This site has plenty of parking, bathrooms, water, picnic and playground facilities, plus a wonderful sandy beach to use as a launch for kayaks.

- At the south end of West Bay there are several options. West End Beach is located at the light at the intersection of US-31 (Division Street) and M-72 (Grandview Parkway). Parking is available, but it may be limited as this is a very popular spot. Bathroom facilities and water are also available.

- Clinch Beach, next to Clinch Marina, is another possibility. Parking, bathrooms and water are available.

- Further east, Sunset Park and Bryant Park both offer parking. Bathrooms are available at Bryant.

DISTANCE/TIME: Of course, this depends on where you put in and where you want to go. We put in at the Elmwood Township Park and paddled to Clinch Marina and back on a gorgeous late September morning. Our trip was about 3.5 miles round trip and took us just under 2 hours.

STRATEGIES: This area is well protected from southerly, westerly and northwesterly winds. Winds from the northeast, east and southeast — though rare — can be problematic on this section.

- A two-vehicle strategy could be used by spotting one vehicle at Bryant Park and the other at the Elmwood Township Park (or vice versa).

FEATURES:

» South of West Bay Marina, you'll see what used to be the dock where coal was delivered by water for the coal-fired power plant. The power plant is long gone — now the Open Space – and the coal dock is now called Discovery Pier.

» This part of West Bay is very protected from most winds and you will be paddling by many moored sailboats. One of them is the *Manitou,* a tall ship that is also a learning vessel. The *Manitou* takes students from schools in northern Michigan on sailing trips to learn about the Bay.

» Next up is the Grand Traverse Yacht Club. Established in 1960, the GTYC eventually moved to its current location on the water in what was once the Manta Mower lawnmower factory.

» Traverse City is the largest city in the 21-county area of northern Michigan. With a population of 14,674, it is the 68th largest city in Michigan. The metropolitan area is considerably larger, with a population of 143,372. Long occupied by Ojibwe and Ottawa peoples, early settlements were located at the base of the Bay, near Clinch Park. In 1847, Henry Boardman arrived and purchased land at the mouth of the Boardman River. In 1851, his sawmill was sold to Hannah, Lay, and Company. Perry Hannah was to become instrumental in the growth and development of Traverse City. Eventually, because of its favorable location and its abundant resources, Traverse City became the largest community in the area, and is today the Cherry Capital of the World. Traverse City is also the gateway to some of the best kayaking to be found anywhere.

» This trip from Greilickville to the Clinch Marina completes the final leg of our series of day-trips around the entire perimeter of the Leelanau Peninsula. In my opinion, these trips are in some of the most accessible and finest stretches of shoreline that you find anywhere. The history, the grandeur of the scenery and the pristine waters can be experienced from no better place than from the cockpit of your kayak — for one mile or all of its 100 miles!

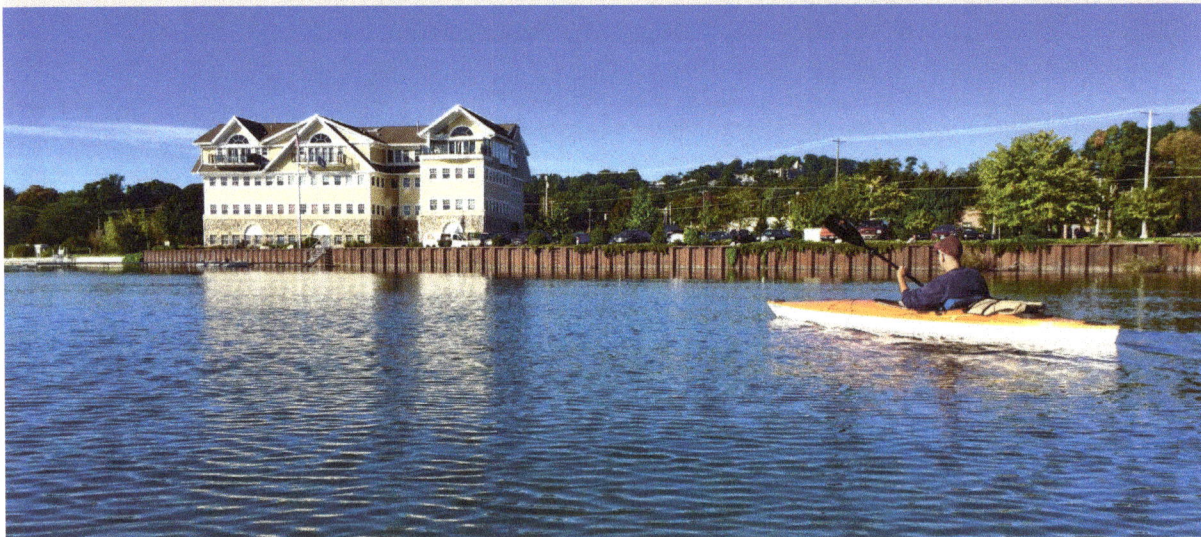

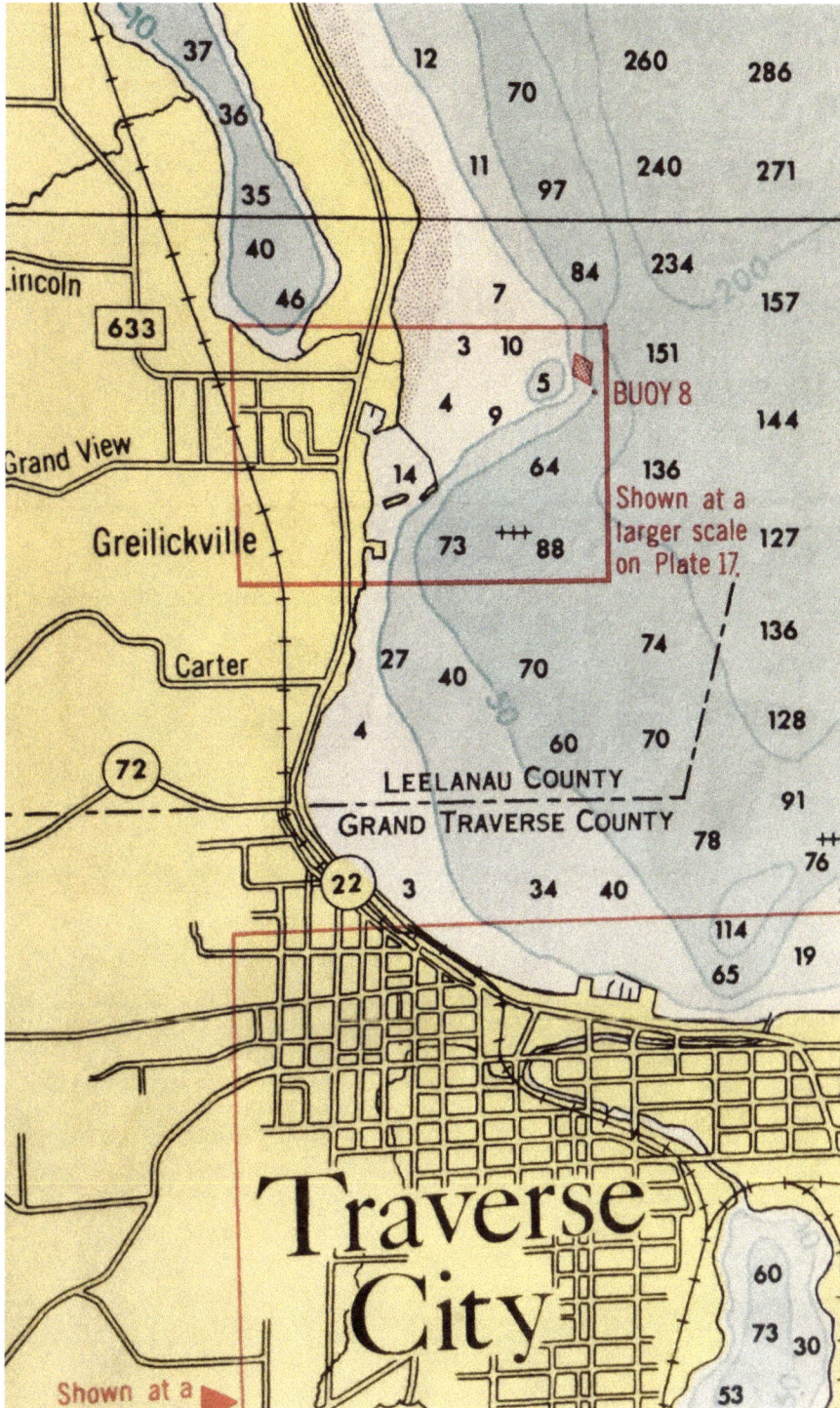

» Greiickville, due to its proximity to Traverse City, is largest populated area and Elmwood Township is the most populous township in Leelanau County.

» At first called Norristown after settlers Seth and Albert Norris who arrived in 1852 and built a grist mill, tannery and brickyard. The brickyard was purchased in 1875 by James W. Markham who switched to steam power instead of horses. Production increased from 200,000 bricks a year to 4 million. Operations ended in 1907.

» Greilickville is named for Godfrey Greilick, an Austrian who came to Norristown from Europe in 1856 with his five sons and built several sawmills, a brewery and a dock. They operated two tugs and three schooners to get lumber from all parts of the Leelanau Peninsula to their facilities. Only Hannah, Lay & Company in Traverse City was bigger. When the railroad came in 1903 the station was given the name Greilickville. Their mill burned down in 1907 and wasn't replaced. The brewery was sold and operated until 1906.

» At the height of the lumbering era, the population of the community was over 300. By 1930 it had fallen to 50. The one lane dirt road was widened and eventually paved. The main route to Suttons Bay was originally more inland (Current County Road 633). Eventually M-22 was built along the shoreline of West Grand Traverse Bay.

Map labels: Lincoln · 633 · Grand View · Greilickville · Carter · 72 · 22 · Traverse City · Shown at a larger scale on Plate 17 · BUOY 8 · LEELANAU COUNTY · GRAND TRAVERSE COUNTY · Shown at a

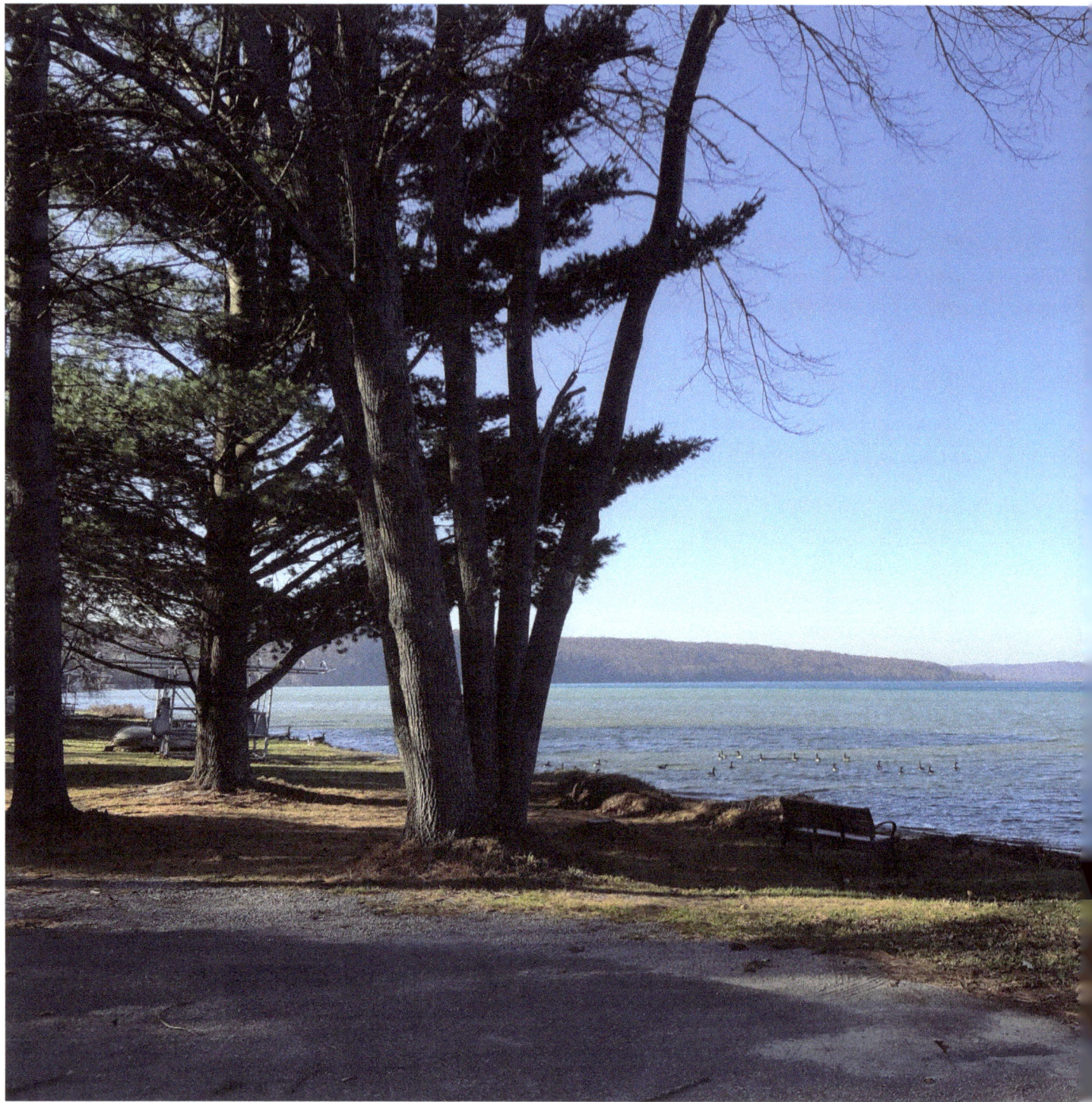

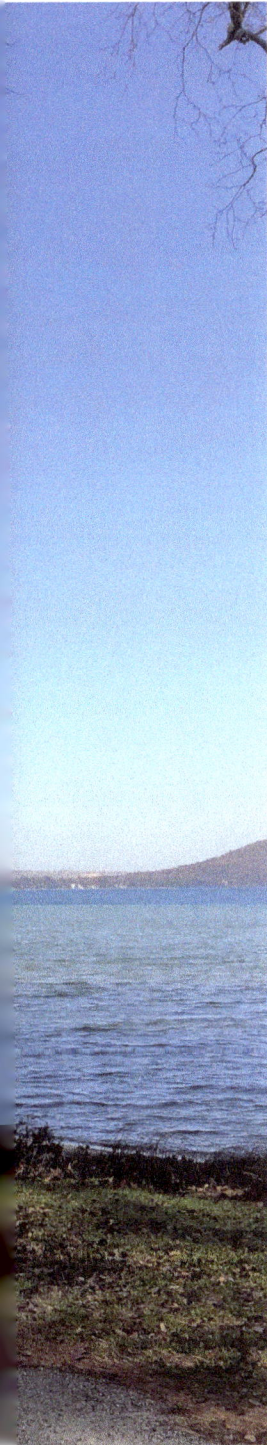

THE INLAND LAKES OF LEELANAU

Kayaking the inland lakes of Leelanau is a delightful alternative to going out on the bigger waters. Larry and I have several times planned to go out on the Big Lake, only to arrive to the sounds of waves pounding the beach. Luckily, the more protected waters of Leelanau's inland lakes are around almost every corner.

There are about 40 named inland lakes in Leelanau County, with public accessibility enough for at least a kayak. In addition, there are three lakes on the two Manitou Islands: Lake Manitou and Tamarack Lake on North Manitou Island and Florence Lake on South Manitou Island.

Some of the inland lakes are large enough for the two-vehicle strategy and a paddle from "A" to "B." There are also many smaller lakes where only one vehicle is needed for a day trip around the shoreline.

The lakes of Leelanau will be presented here in a general direction from west to east. The shoreline lengths and areas of the lakes in this book are used by permission from Jim Stamm and his book, *A Guide to the Rivers and Lakes of Grand Traverse and Leelanau Counties, Michigan*. Stamm's book provides very good detailed information on how to access many of Leelanau's inland lakes, as well as additional information on the rivers.

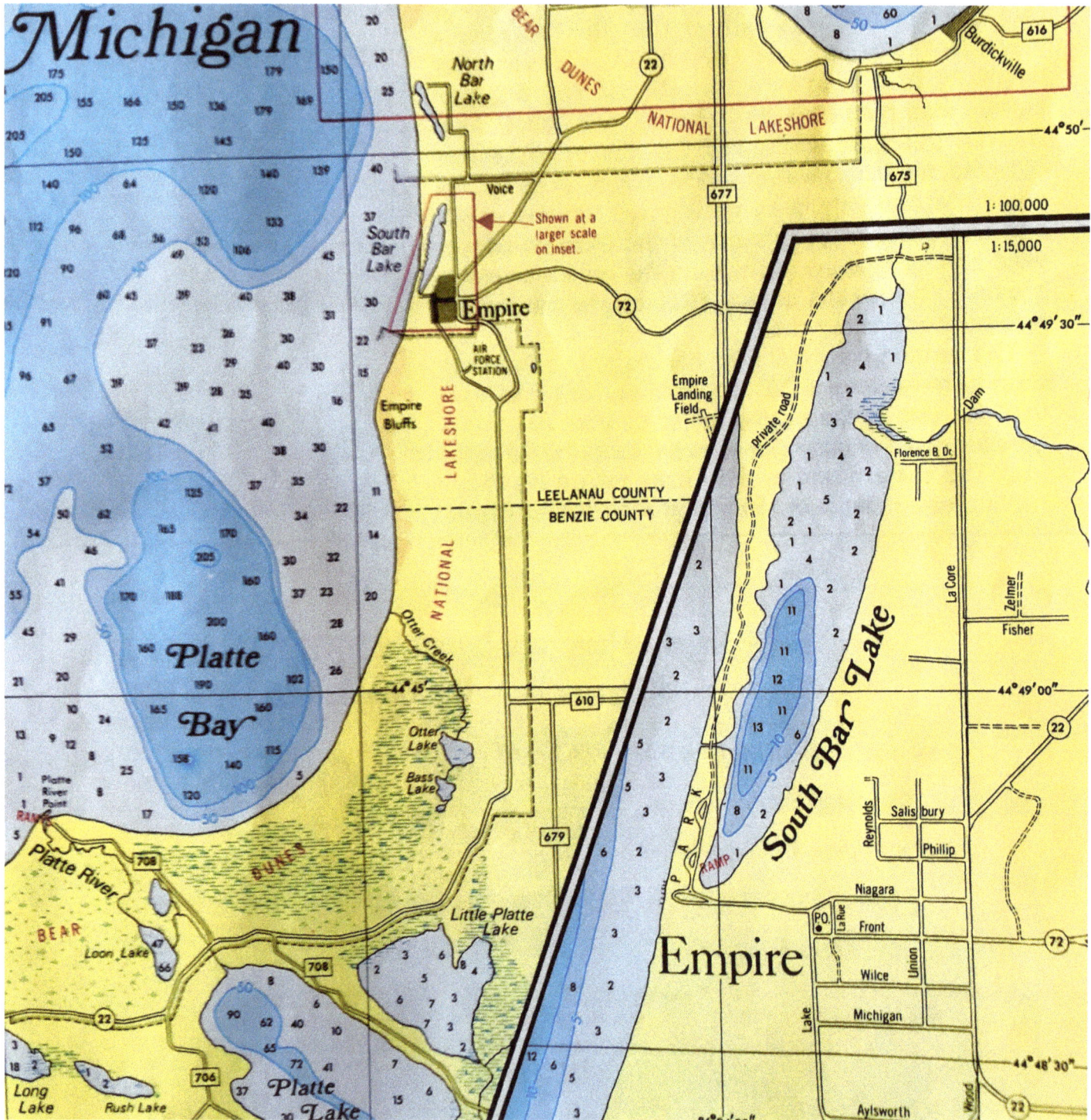

Michigan

North Bar Lake

BEAR DUNES

22

NATIONAL LAKESHORE

44°50'

Burdickville

616

South Bar Lake

Voice

677

675

1:100,000

Shown at a larger scale on inset.

1:15,000

Empire

AIR FORCE STATION

72

44°49'30"

Empire Bluffs

Empire Landing Field

private road

Florence B. Dr.

LAKESHORE

LEELANAU COUNTY
BENZIE COUNTY

South Bar Lake

La Core

Zelmer

Fisher

NATIONAL

Otter Creek

44°45'

44°49'00"

22

610

Platte

Bay

Otter Lake

Bass Lake

P A R K

RAMP

Reynolds

Salisbury

Phillip

Niagara

PO.

LaRue

Front

Empire

Platte River Point

RAMP

Platte River

708

679

Little Platte Lake

Wilce

Union

BEAR

Loon Lake

708

Lake

Michigan

72

22

706

Long Lake

Rush Lake

Platte Lake

Aylsworth

Wood

44°48'30"

22

SOUTH BAR LAKE

This beautiful, smaller lake is one of the best things about Empire, Michigan. It is located right in Lake Michigan Beach Park and is one of the park's finest features.

LOCATION: South Bar Lake is in the village of Empire, 24 miles west of Traverse City.

ACCESS: South Bar Lake can be accessed at Lake Michigan Beach Park, which is on Niagara Street, just northwest of the main business district in Empire (Lake Street). The park has plenty of amenities, including parking (a parking fee is required), a small dock, a paved launch and bathroom facilities.

INFORMATION:

» This is a small 81-acre lake with a shoreline of 2.4 miles.

» South Bar Lake is deeper on the southern end (some areas are around 10 feet) and shallower on the northern end (only around 5 feet).

» The lake is fed by several small streams on its north and east boundaries and it has an outlet to Lake Michigan that goes over a small dam.

» The slabs of wood visible on the bottom the lake on the western and northern parts of the lake are echoes of the busy sawmill days of early Empire."

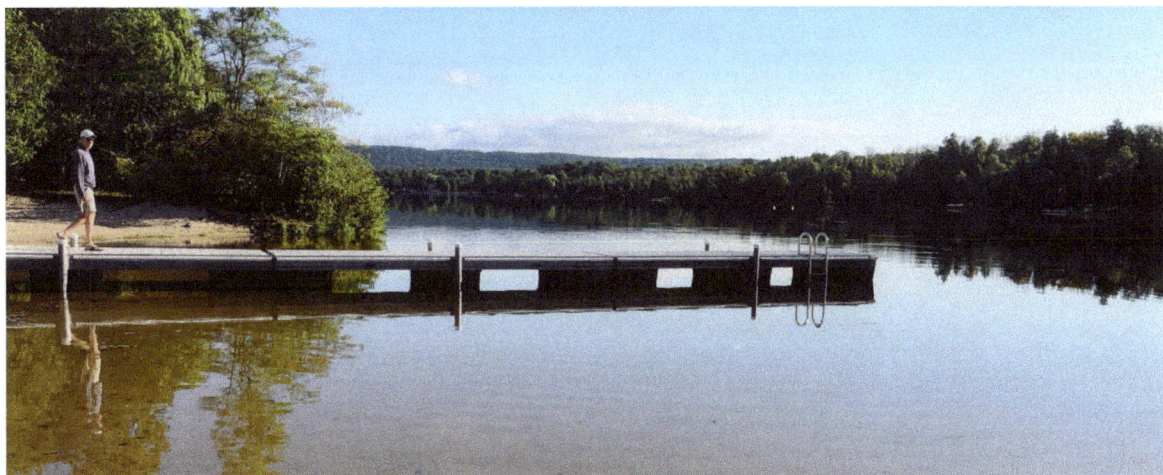

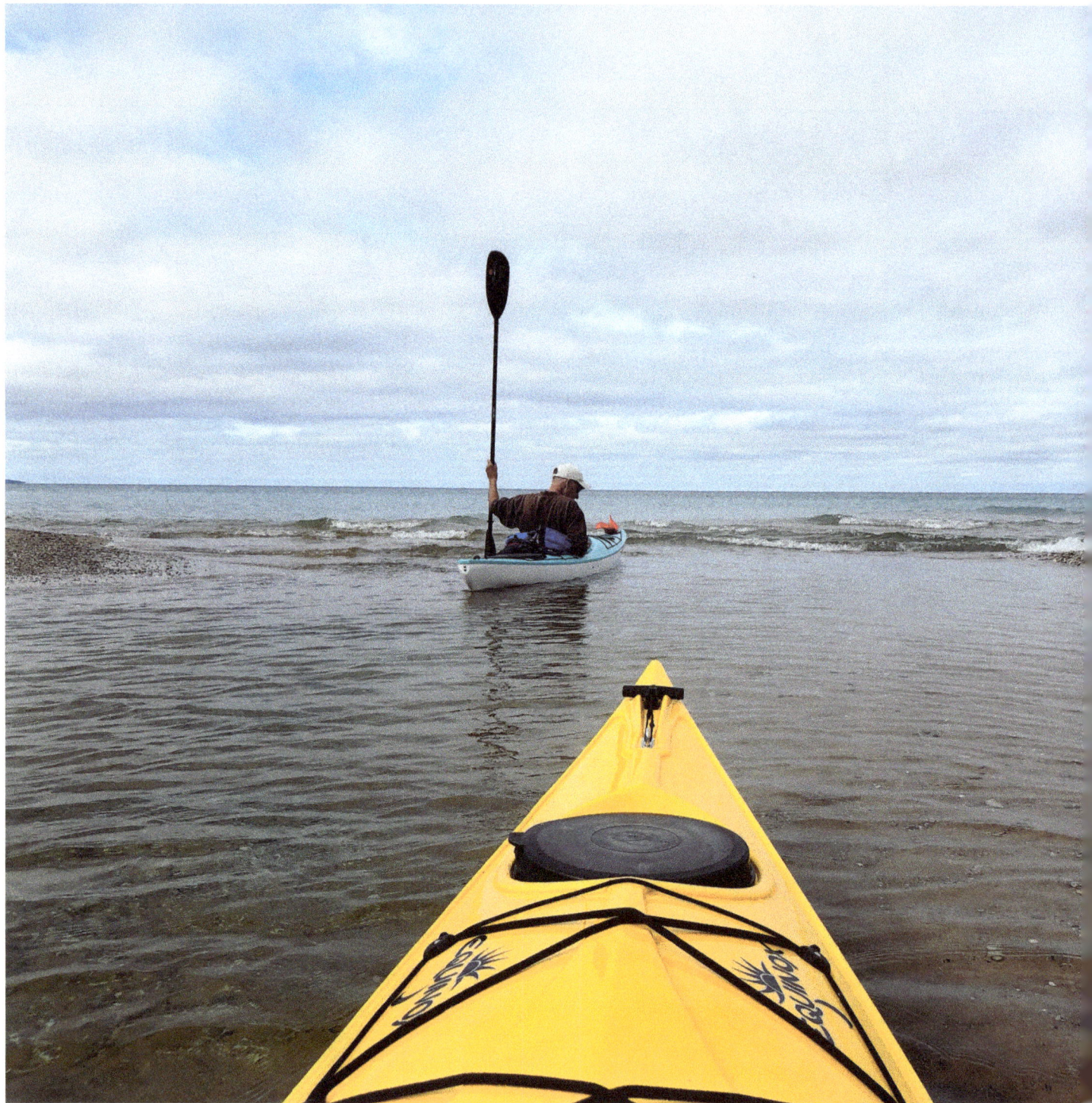

NORTH BAR LAKE

North Bar Lake is a local favorite. This hidden gem is a bit off the beaten path, but is well worth the effort to visit it.

LOCATION: North Bar Lake is located between Empire and Glen Haven, just south of the Pierce Stocking Trail in the Sleeping Bear Dunes National Lakeshore. It is about 25 miles west of Traverse City.

ACCESS: There is a parking area that requires a National Park Pass just east of North Bar Lake. It's a short walk from the parking area to a spot to put in. The park is located west of M-22, and can be found by taking Voice Road to North Bar Lake Road to Larohr Road.

INFORMATION:

» North Bar Lake is a small, 30-acre, elongated lake, similar to South Bar Lake. It has a shoreline of 1.5 miles.

» This little lake seemed to be consistently shallow, not exceeding 10 feet.

» Although there are no tributaries showing on the North Bar Lake map, there is an outlet to Lake Michigan about 500 feet in length that has looked different every single time that I've seen it. The channel varies, depending on the levels of Lake Michigan and North Bar Lake and the actions of the sand along Lake Michigan.

COMMENTS:

» A National Park pass is required.

» This is a beautiful lake with marshes, woods and sand dunes along its shore. It is closed to all motorized boats. On hot days, expect a large number of adults and children enjoying the beach and water.

» A day trip to this little gem of a lake can include a paddle on a small lake, a paddle in Lake Michigan, then a swim in either lake. Many people who visit this spot take a short beach walk to the base of "The Climb," at the lookout on the Pierce Stocking Trail — one of the most popular features of the Sleeping Bear Dunes National Lakeshore.

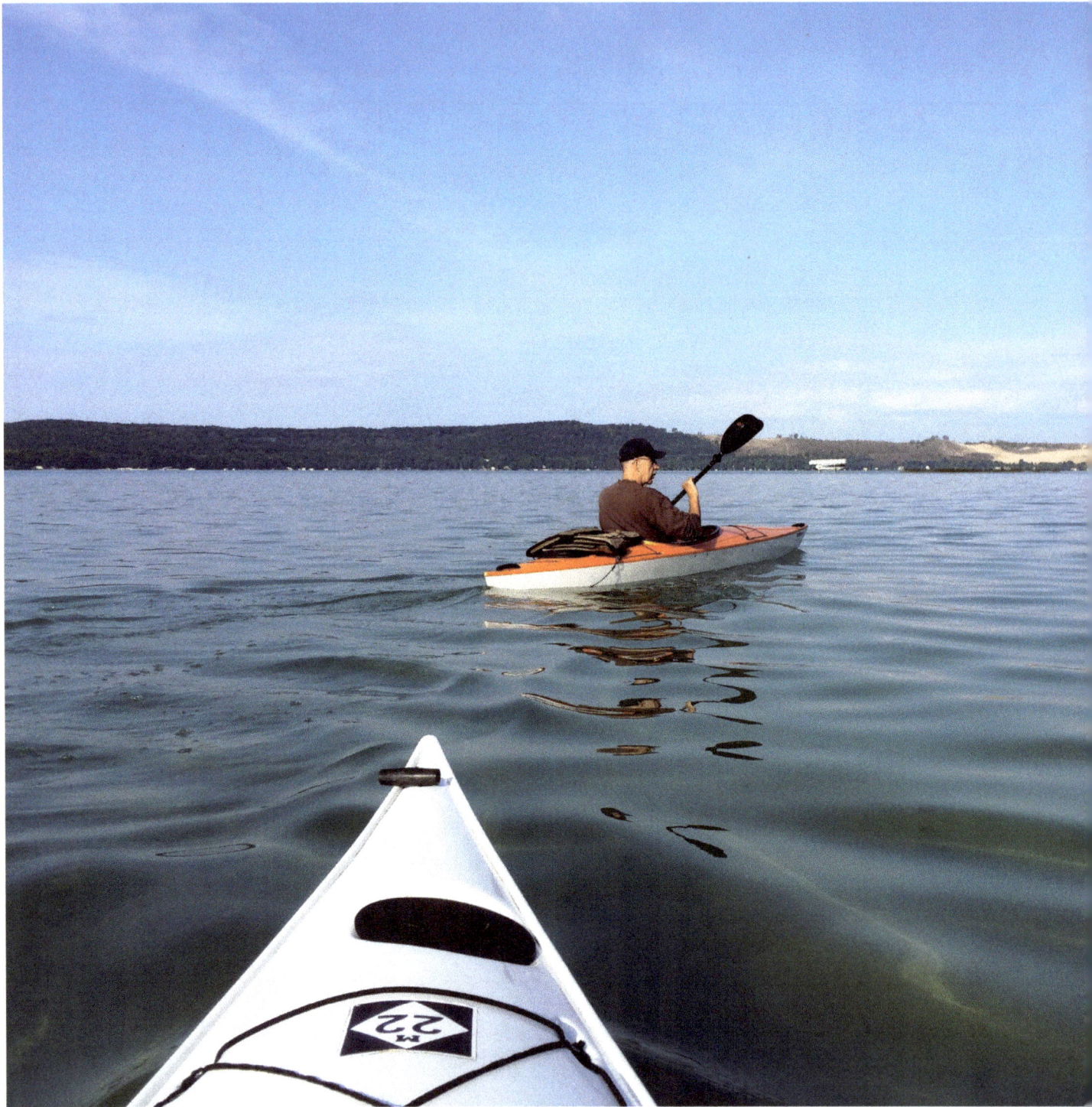

LITTLE GLEN LAKE

The views of the "Sleeping Bear Dunes"— especially "The Climb," to the west of Little Glen Lake — are outstanding from the perspective of a kayak. Alligator Hill to the north, The Narrow's bridge to the east and the wooded hills to the south make this a lake with a setting like no other.

LOCATION: This gem is located southwest of Glen Arbor and directly west of Big Glen Lake. M-22 goes along much of its southern shore, and crosses The Narrows on its eastern edge. Little Glen is about 20 miles north and west of Traverse City.

ACCESS: The best access point is the DNR launch on Day Forest Road, on the north shore of Little Glen. This launch is less than a half-mile from M-22 and The Narrows. There is parking, a hard surface launch, a dock and restrooms. One of the times we launched from here, the parking lot was full and we needed to park on Day Forest Road.

INFORMATION:

» Little Glen Lake is a medium- to large-sized lake. It is an all-sports lake of 1,400 acres and a 6.4 mile shoreline.

» Little Glen Lake is much shallower than its neighbor, Big Glen Lake. Little Glen is shallow along its shore and its western half (averaging 3 feet). Towards The Narrows, it averages 13 feet in the center of the lake.

» The Michigan DNR fishing map shows that there are several small spring tributaries flowing into the lake on its southern shore. Little Glen is connected to Big Glen Lake at its eastern end, at The Narrows, and this is the only outlet.

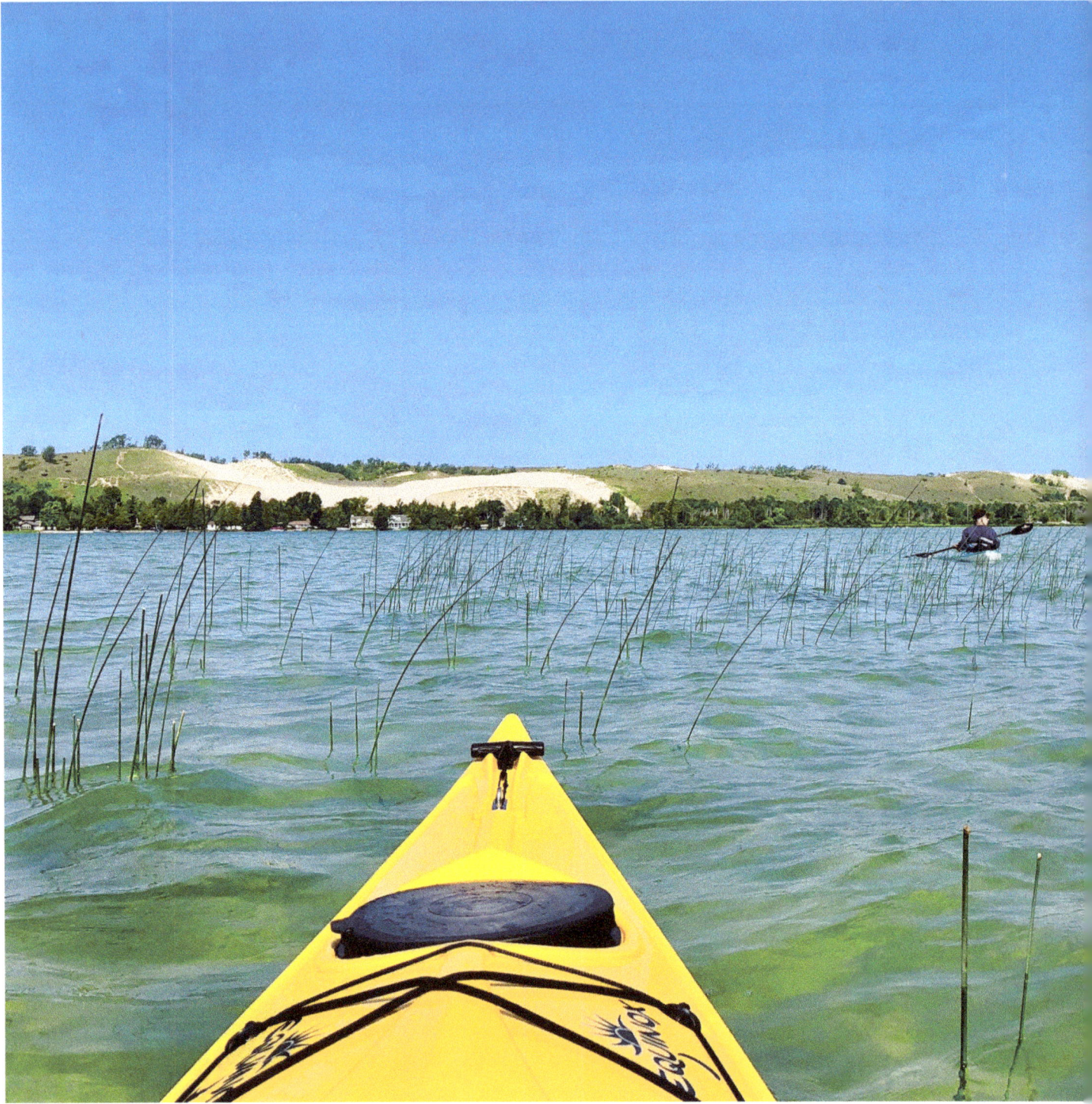

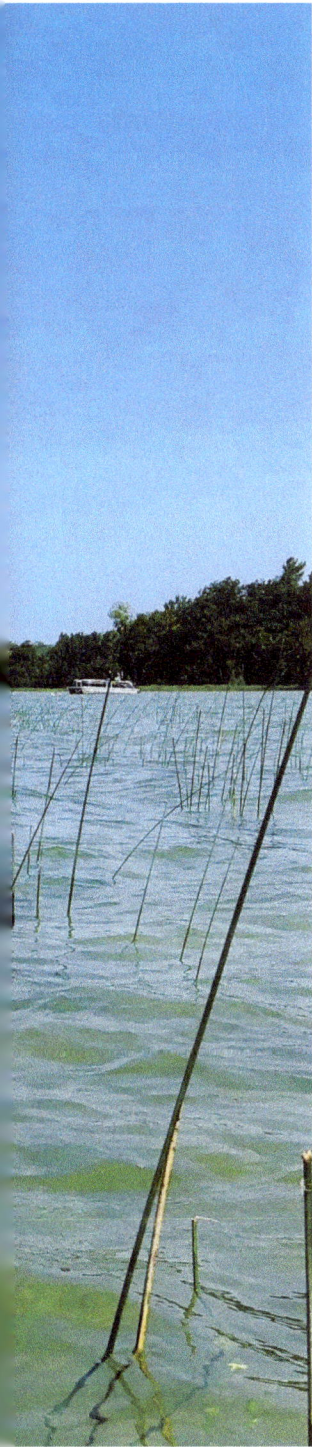

COMMENTS:

» This oval-shaped lake offers a great paddle around its shore. The views of the sand dunes to the west, Alligator Hill to the north and the wooded hills to the south are about as good as you can get anywhere. The homes and cottages along the shore are also interesting to look at.

» Thousands of years ago, this lake was formerly an embayment of the larger and higher Lake Algonquin, which preceded Lake Michigan (and the last ice age). Other lakes in the region, like Crystal Lake in Benzie County and North and South Bar Lakes, were also formed when they were cut off from Lake Algonquin by sand moving steadily along their shorelines as the old lake receded.

» This area was hit by a devastating wind event on August 2, 2015. Winds estimated at up to 100 miles an hour knocked down countless trees, damaged homes, boats and hoists. A month later, Larry and I kayaked the lake and talked to a homeowner on the west end who said winds pushed the water away from her shore, leaving her boat hoist and dock high and dry for a few minutes! A year later we still heard chainsaws clearing fallen and damaged trees from this event.

» I have read that Little Glen was once as deep as Big Glen, but has been filling up with sand for thousands of years. If this is a sign that it will be filling up completely in another thousand years, you better plan your trip here right away!

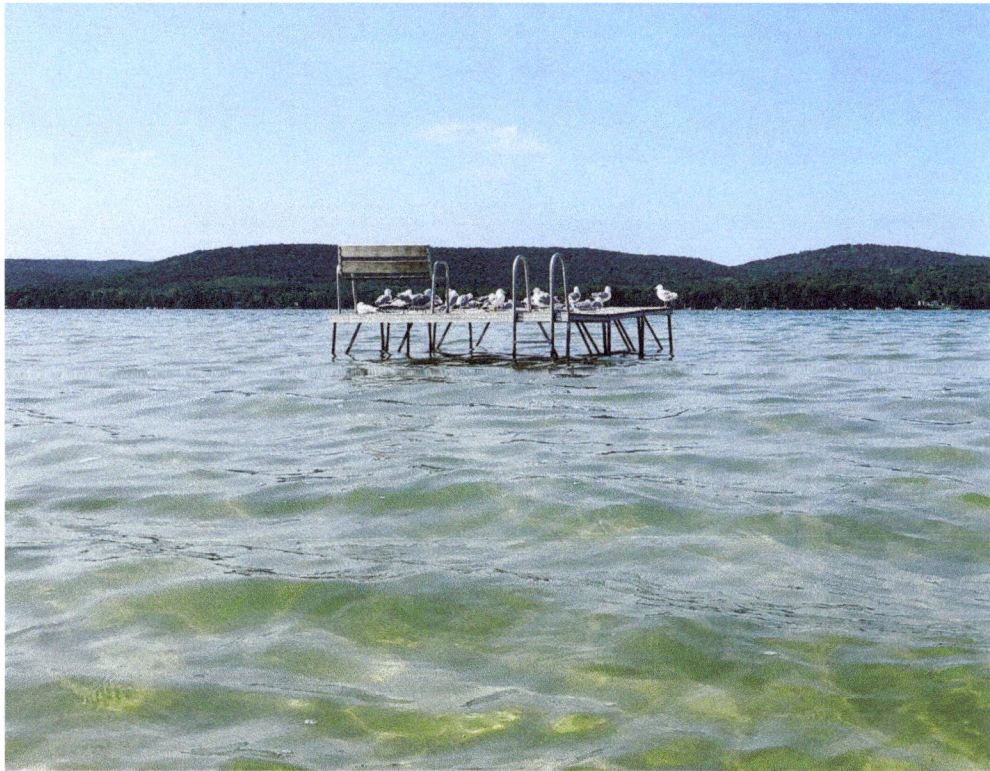

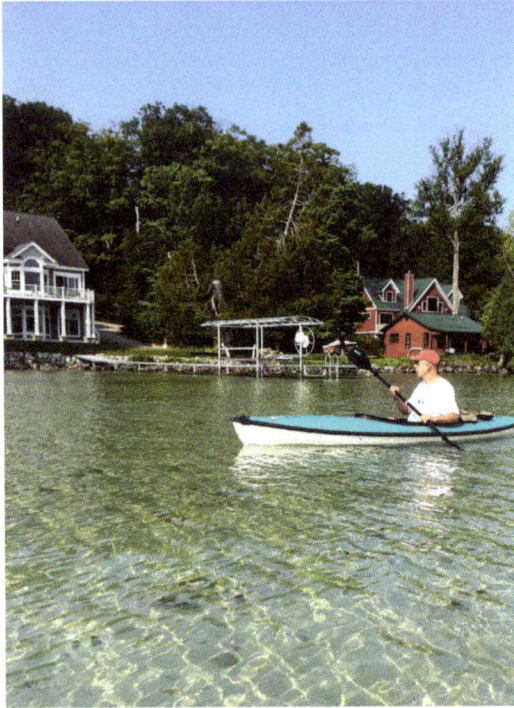
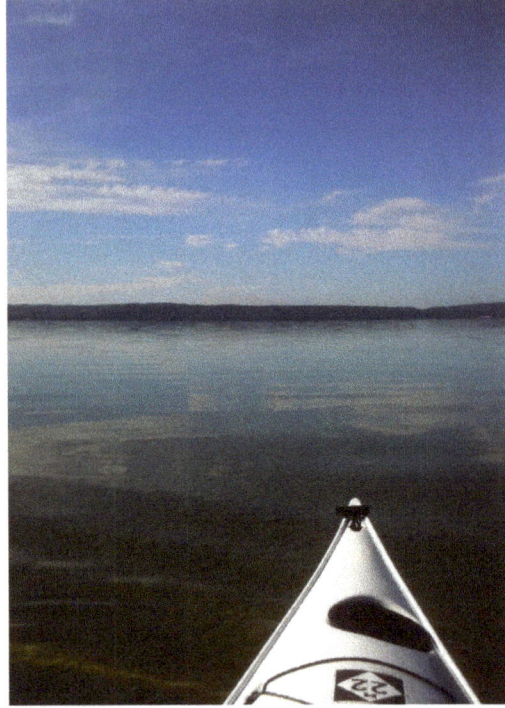
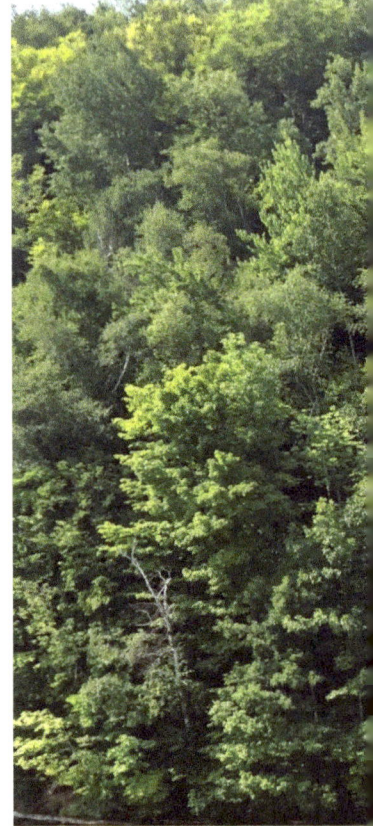
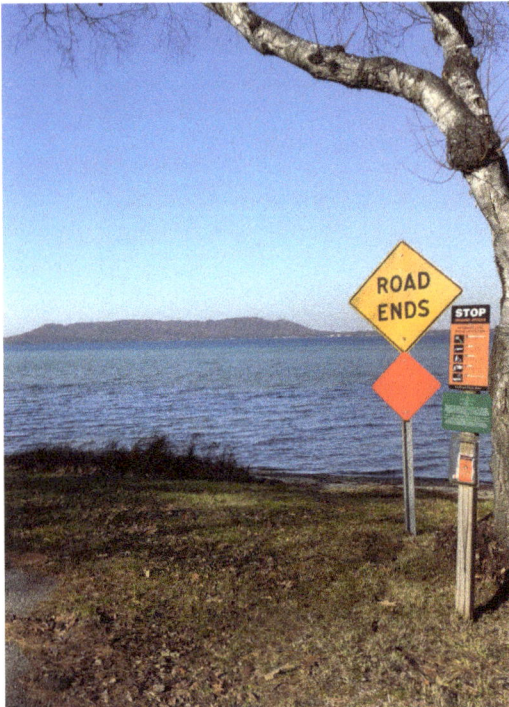
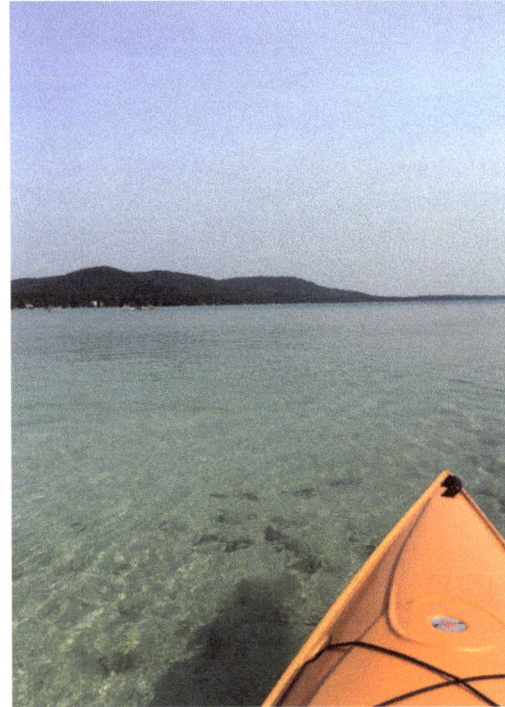
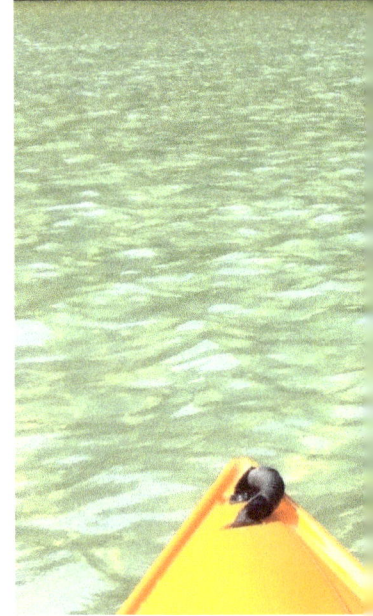

BIG GLEN LAKE

Big Glen is big enough that you can spend several days exploring. This lake is one of Michigan's "must paddle" destinations. There are great water, great views and some spectacular real estate!

LOCATION: Big Glen Lake is about a mile southeast of Glen Arbor, just east of Little Glen Lake and about 20 miles northwest of Traverse City.

ACCESS: For our trips to Big Glen Lake, we have used the Little Glen Lake access on Day Forest Road, then paddled under the bridge and into the lake.

- We have also used the Old Settlers Campgrounds on the southeastern side of the lake. The park is just north of Burdickville and the intersection of Burdickville Road (County Road 616) and Dunns Farm Road (County Road 675). The campground has plenty of parking, a dock, a small inclined path leading to a landing and restrooms.

- Other possible access sites include county roads that dead end at the lake — perfect for a kayak launch.

- On the north shore, there's access next to Glen Craft Marina at the end of Lake Street and less than a mile from the central business district in Glen Arbor. There is limited parking here.

- For a southern access, drive to the end of Agnew Street, just north of Burdickville. This street is near the Trattoria Funistrada and La Becasse restaurants.

INFORMATION:

» Big Glen is the second largest inland lake in Leelanau County at 4,865 acres. (Only South Lake Leelanau is larger). Big Glen Lake is oval-shaped with a shoreline of 10.8 miles.

» Big Glen is the deepest of all of the lakes in Leelanau County. The deepest areas reach 130 feet.

» The major inlet is the water from Little Glen that flows into Big Glen via The Narrows.

» There are several other streams and spring tributaries that feed Big Glen Lake. Hadlem Creek flows into the lake on its southern shore. Tiny Brooks Lake flows into the lake just north of Old Settler's Park. And water from the even smaller Brooks Lake flows into Big Glen on the eastern side, just north of Old Settler's Park.

» The only outlet from Big Glen Lake is the water that empties into Lake Michigan by way of the flow into Fisher Lake and then into the Crystal River.

COMMENTS:

» Big Glen Lake has been called the most beautiful lake in the USA, and it's hard to argue with that. Set between wooded hills and sandy dunes, its spectacular water can be a Caribbean blue-green color.

» Two of my favorite spots to view this lake are Inspiration Point, on the south side of the lake, and Miller Hill to its east. The view from Inspiration Point, high above the lake, offers views of Lake Michigan and the Manitous in the distance. The view from Miller Hill looks west and includes Tucker and Fisher Lakes, and the Sleeping Bear Dunes in the far distance.

» Burdickville was another one of the many Leelanau lumber towns to develop in the 1800s, only to see their fortunes wane as the source of lumber dwindled.

» One of the interesting stories about Glen Lake is about the 32-foot wooden steamer named *Rescue*. In the late 1800s, Glen Lake didn't have a great number of steam ships for ferrying tourists and locals like Lake Leelanau, but it did have *Rescue*. The boat was owned and operated by Ralph Dorsey — at least until 1914, when he intentionally scuttled it by hacking holes in the bottom of the boat with an axe. Mr. Dorsey made it back to shore, but the boat sank in one of the deepest parts of Big Glen, where it sits today. What drove him to sink his boat and his livelihood is not clear, but theories range from his mental state to worries about his finances to losing *Rescue* in a game of cards.

» Big Glen has some of the most coveted — and costly — lakeshore property in the entire region.

» Glen Lake was originally called Bear Lake because of the numerous bears in the nearby forests and the common encounters the bears had with the early settlers.

» In the 1860's there was a plan to cut a canal from Glen Lake to Lake Michigan was proposed, but the idea was never completed.

» In 1871 the first bridge was built at the narrows, a wooden one. It had a lift span to allow a tug and its scow to pass through with lumber or other goods.

» Around 1899 J.O. Nesson built two sawmills, one on the northeast shore of Glen Lake and the other across the lake at Burdickville and also built a railroad tramway from the lake to shore of Sleeping Bear Bay just east of Glen Arbor. It was in operation until 1907. Decades later the steam locomotive was used as a tourist attraction at Clinch Park in Traverse City.

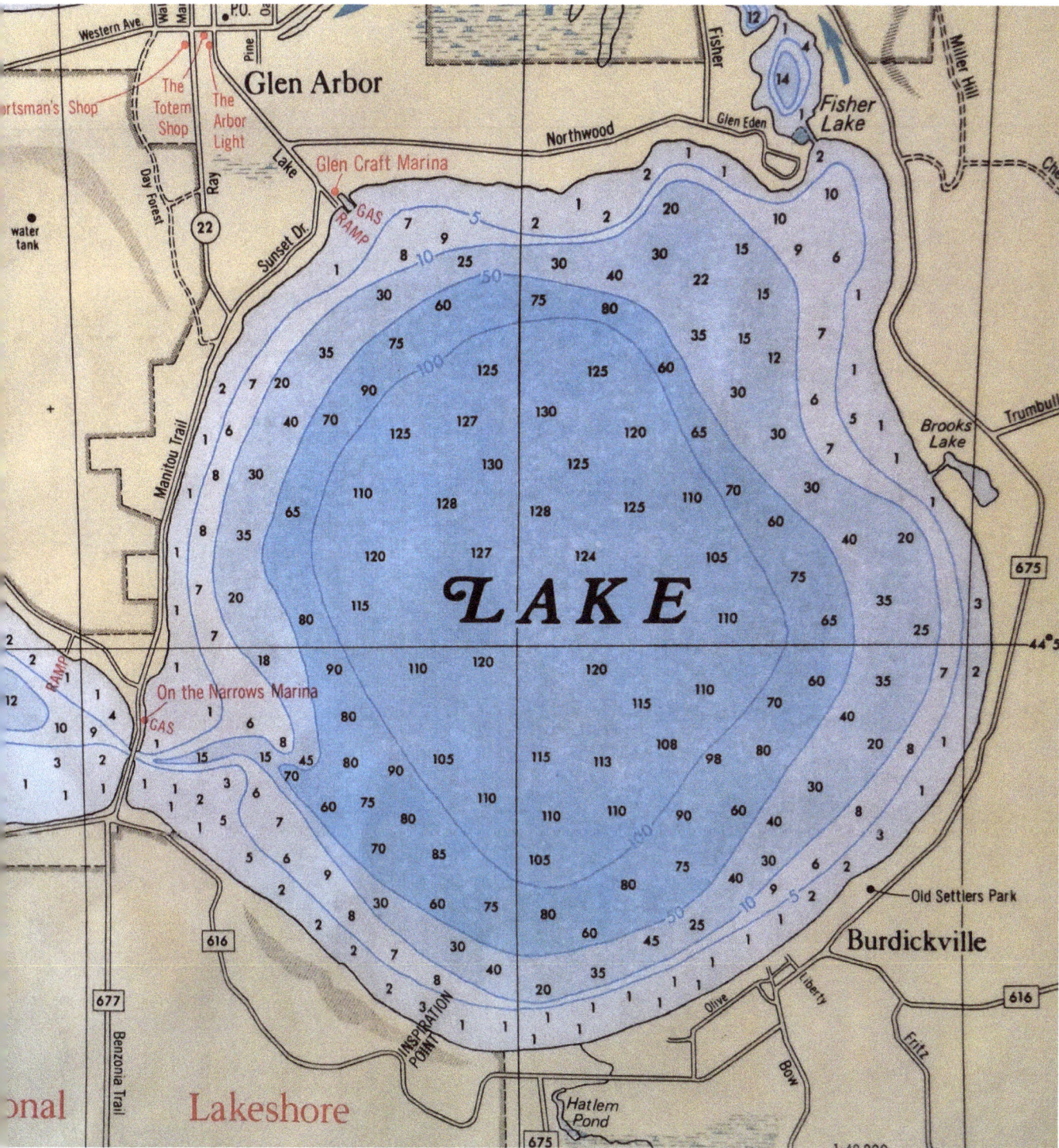

Glen Arbor

Western Ave.

P.O.

Pine

Oak

The Sportsman's Shop
The Totem Shop
The Arbor Light

Day Forest

Ray

Lake

22

water tank

Sunset Dr.

Glen Craft Marina

GAS
RAMP

Northwood

Glen Eden

Fisher

Fisher Lake

Miller Hill

14

12

Manitou Trail

LAKE

Brooks Lake

Trumbull

675

On the Narrows Marina

GAS

RAMP

12

44° 5

Old Settlers Park

Burdickville

616

616

677

Benzonia Trail

616

INSPIRATION POINT

Olive

Bow

Liberty

Fritz

Hatlem Pond

675

Lakeshore

onal

1:40,000

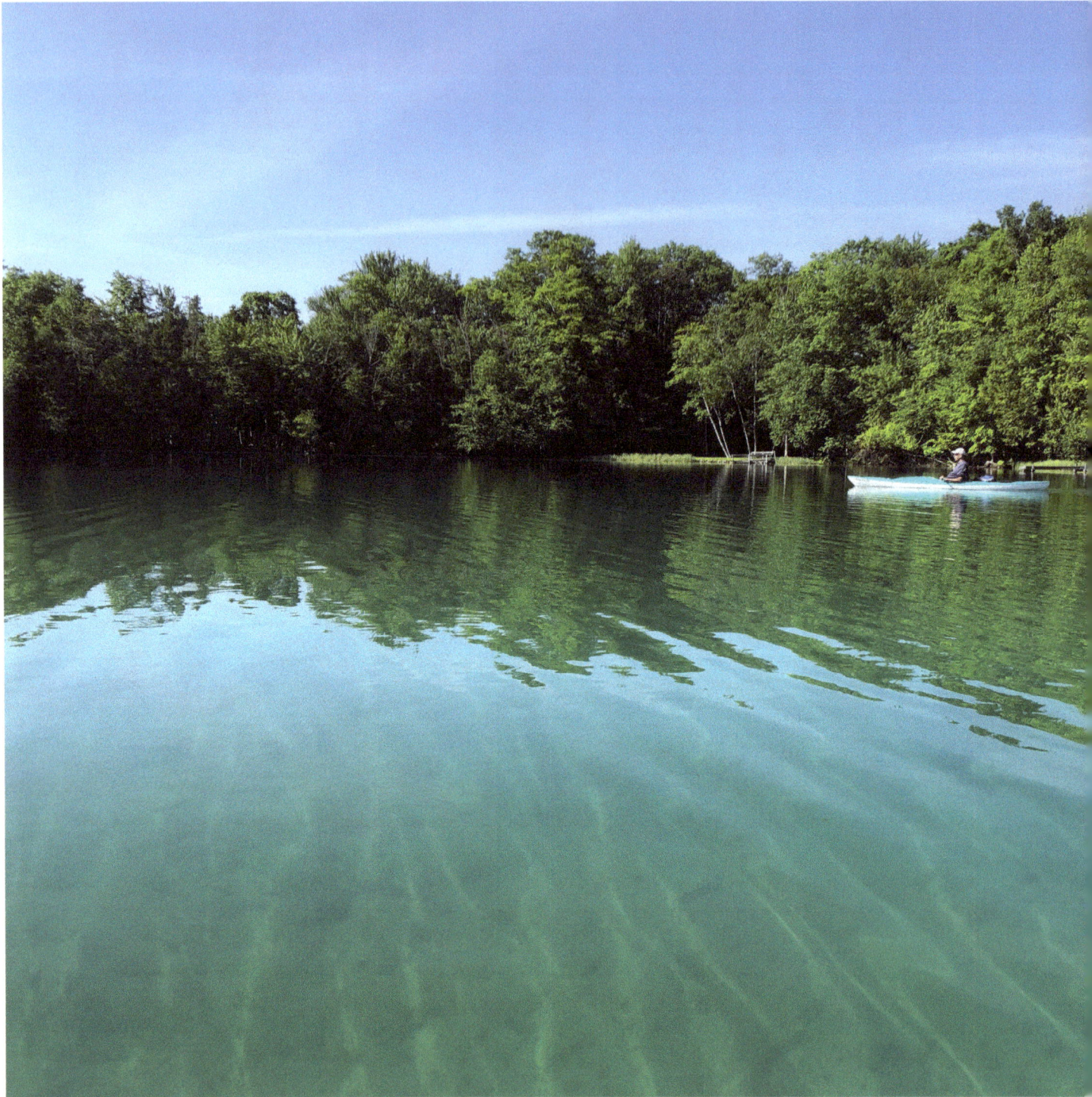

FISHER LAKE

Fisher Lake is a little lake connected to Big Glen Lake. There are lots of trees and vegetation and some nice homes and cottages on its shores. A small finger of a peninsula juts into Fisher Lake, making for two sections. Unfortunately, the day we paddled this lake my camera's battery died. Trust me that this is a beautiful lake.

LOCATION: Fisher Lake is located southeast of Glen Arbor and immediately north of Big Glen Lake. It is about 24 miles northwest of Traverse City.

ACCESS: We paddled Fisher Lake by putting in our kayaks at the Old Settler's Campgrounds on Big Glen and entering Fisher Lake from the south. In June of 2018 we put in at the northwest tip of the lake where Fisher Road intersects with Dunn's Farm Road (County Road 675). We parked in the Crystal River Sleeping Bear Dunes National Lakeshore parking lot and launched across the street by the culvert where Fisher Lake flows into the Crystal River.

INFORMATION:

» Fisher Lake is on the smaller side, with an area of 52 acres and a shoreline of only 1.8 miles. It is somewhat divided by a peninsula that juts into the lake from its western shore and creates two sections — the much larger is to the south. If you put in at either Old Settler's Park or from Lake Street, the distance of the paddle increases.

» Fisher Lake's deepest part is about 14 feet in its southern section and about 12 feet in its northern part.

» The major inlet is the water that flows into Fisher Lake from a channel in Big Glen Lake. There is also a stream that enters the lake on its northern edge from nearby Tucker Lake. The only outlet from Fisher Lake is the Crystal River that flows from its northern shore, past Glen Arbor and on into Lake Michigan at the Homestead Resort.

» Fisher Lake is named for John E. Fisher, who came to the area in 1853 and owned the land surrounding the lake. Fisher also named the Crystal River because he was so impressed by the clarity of its water.

COMMENTS:

» Locals often describe the two sections of this lake as Big Fisher Lake and Little Fisher Lake. The bigger, southern section has a depth of 15 feet in its center. The smaller, northern section has a maximum depth of 12 feet.

» We saw lots of small and large fish on our paddle on this lake — and some great blue herons looking for a meal.

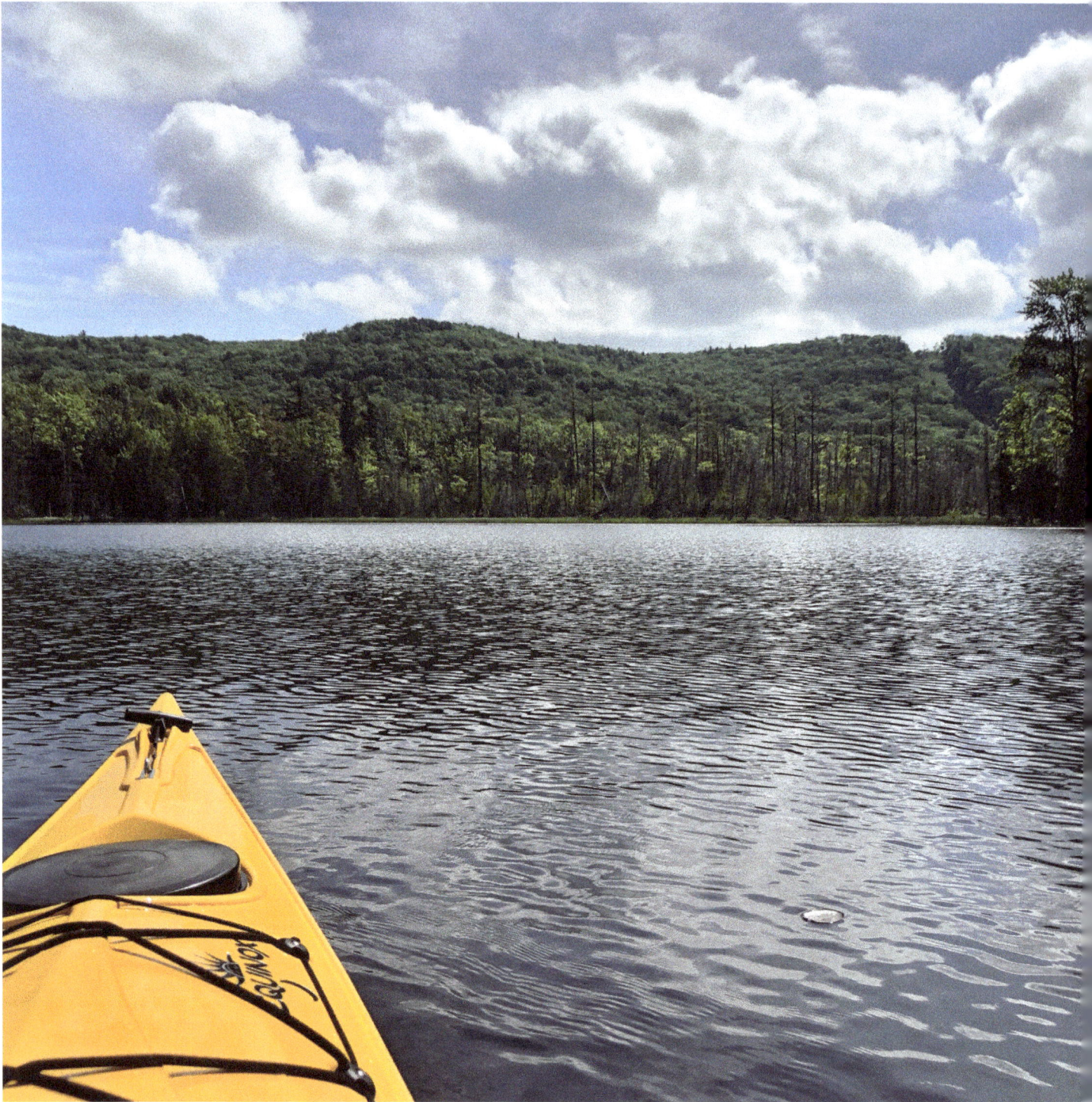

TUCKER LAKE

We visited this lake on June 12, 2018 on a day we also visited nearby Fisher and Shell Lakes. We had Tucker Lake all to ourselves—other than more dragonflies than I could count. The lake itself has no developments around it and is a great place for a quiet paddle. We saw a beaver house and many, many beautiful lily pads in bloom. Miller Hill looms over this little lake and is a great scenic backdrop. This would be a wonderful place to paddle in autumn with the trees on Miller Hill in their fall colors.

LOCATION: Tucker Lake is located just north of Fisher Lake and Glen Lake, east of Glen Arbor. It is about 26 miles from Traverse City.

ACCESS: There is a landing on the western side of the lake, off Westman Road, near the intersection of Dunns Farm Road (County Road 675) and Fisher Road. The road leading to the landing is gravel, and parking is limited and requires a National Park Pass. There are no bathroom facilities.

INFORMATION:

» Tucker Lake is a small lake of under 20 acres and has a shoreline of 0.6 miles.

» The Tucker Lake map shows several small inlets on the northwest and west sides. There is a tributary that connects Tucker Lake to nearby Fisher Lake.

COMMENTS:

» This little lake really appeals to the paddler who wants to enjoy nature and "get away from the crowds." Miller Hill, to the east, provides a beautiful backdrop to the unspoiled vegetation, dead trees and stumps on its shore.

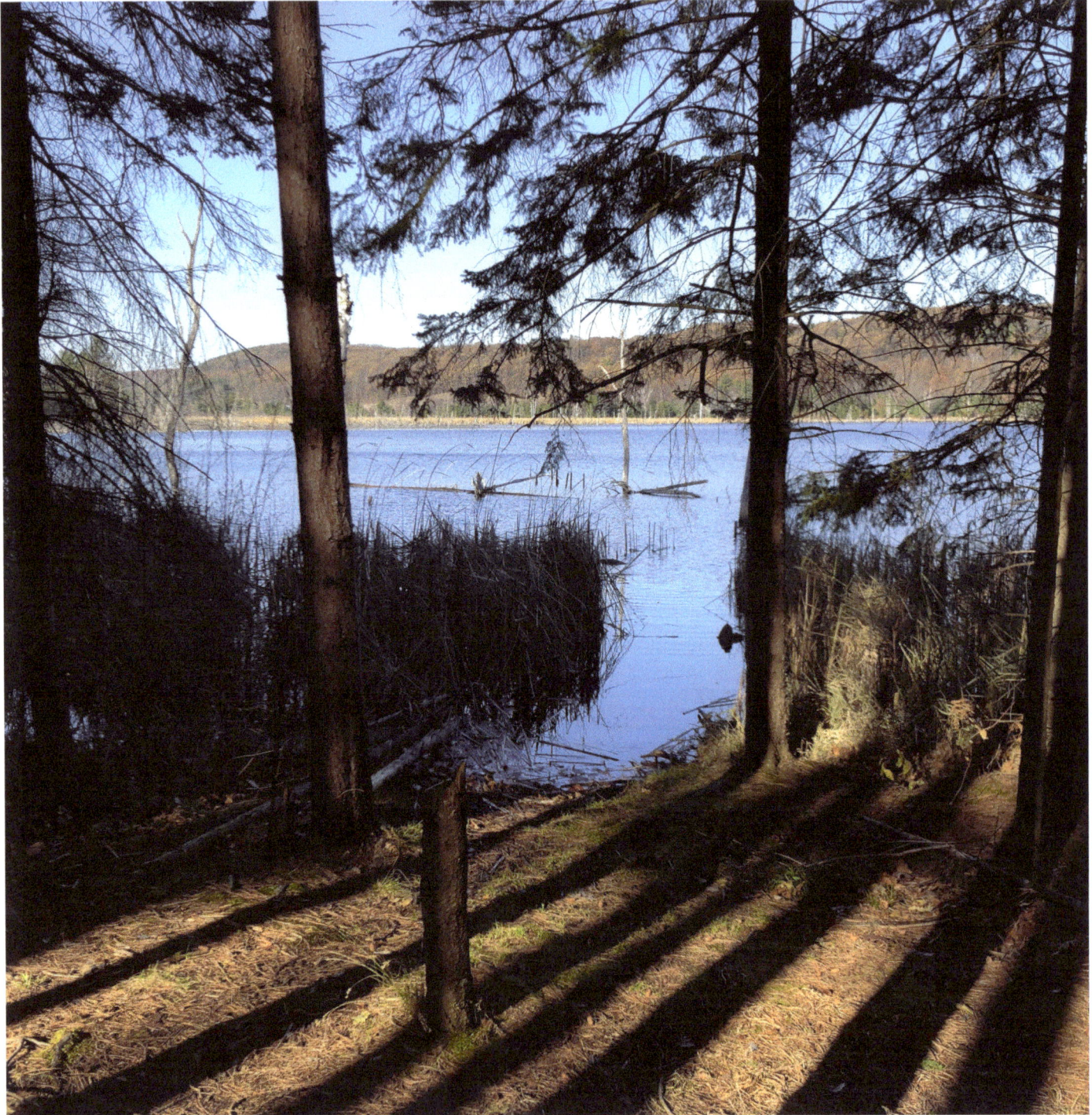

NARADA LAKE

This gem includes a beaver dam at its east end.

LOCATION: Narada Lake is located east of Port Oneida and southeast of Pyramid Point, between Wheeler Road and Bohemian Road — you can see it from M-22.

ACCESS: The access point is located east of the guard rail on M-22. There's a footpath just east of the wooden bike/hiking bridge that extends over some of Narada Lake's wetlands. You will have to park by the side of the highway.

INFORMATION:

» Narada Lake, at 35 acres, is slightly larger than North Bar Lake and has a shoreline of 1.2 miles.

» There are no inlets to Narada Lake. There is one outlet on its eastern side that often includes a beaver dam. This stream flows into Shalda Creek, and then into Lake Michigan.

COMMENTS:

» There is an abandoned farm at the eastern edge of the lake, which is now part of the Sleeping Bear Dunes National Lakeshore.

» It's estimated that the beavers have raised the lake up to 8 feet. Be wary of submerged stumps, trees and vegetation.

» This is prime bald eagle territory!

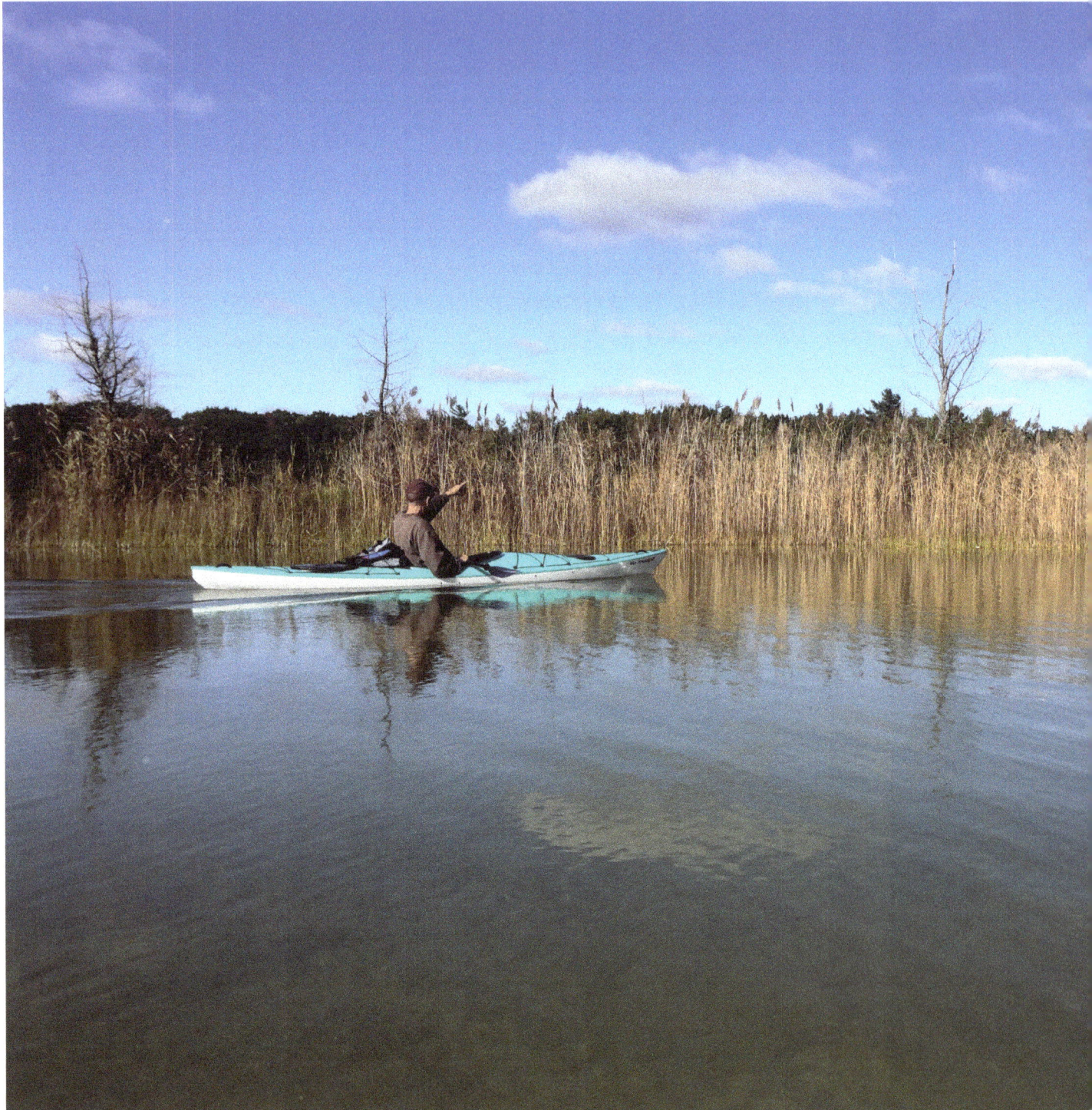

SHELL LAKE

I am amazed that there are so many quiet, pristine and natural lakes so close to the urban environment of Traverse City. Shell Lake is one of them. It takes a little effort to get to, but with its partial views of nearby Pyramid Point, the sounds of waves on nearby Lake Michigan and the beauty of unspoiled nature, it's so worth it. Shell Lake requires a National Park Pass. No motorized watercraft are allowed.

LOCATION: Shell Lake is northeast of Glen Arbor.

ACCESS: We accessed Shell Lake at a carry-in, sandy area at the end of a two-track road. To reach that two-track, go to the end of Bohemian Road (County Road 669) and take Lake Michigan Road 2.3 miles west to an intersection. Go left about 0.2 miles to another intersection, and take the two-track a short distance to a turnaround. The beach is at the turnaround. Parking is very limited, but there's usually little competition for spots. Good luck.

- There were signs that the park was developing a new access on the northwest side of the lake. Be ready to use this improved location.

INFORMATION:

» Shell Lake is a small- to medium-sized lake with a 2.2 mile shoreline. At around 90 acres, it is a little larger than South Bar Lake. Much of the lake was around 3 to 5 feet deep, with a few spots reaching 12 to 15 feet in depth.

» There are no inlets or outlets.

COMMENTS:

» The day we were there we saw a few fishermen casting from shore. After they left, we didn't see another person the rest of the day.

» At the southwestern edge of the lake there was an old weathered dock and some pilings. The Michigan DNR map for Shell Lake shows this as a "Boat Livery." The story that goes with that livery would be interesting to know.

» It took us under an hour to go around this pretty little lake, but it was one of my favorite paddles of the summer. The serenity and the beauty were well worth the effort to get to and on the lake.

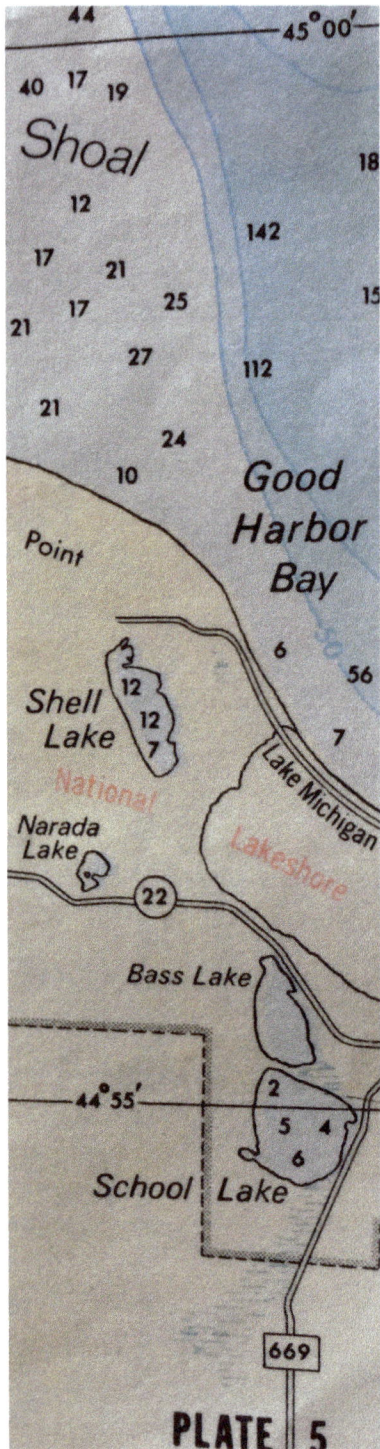

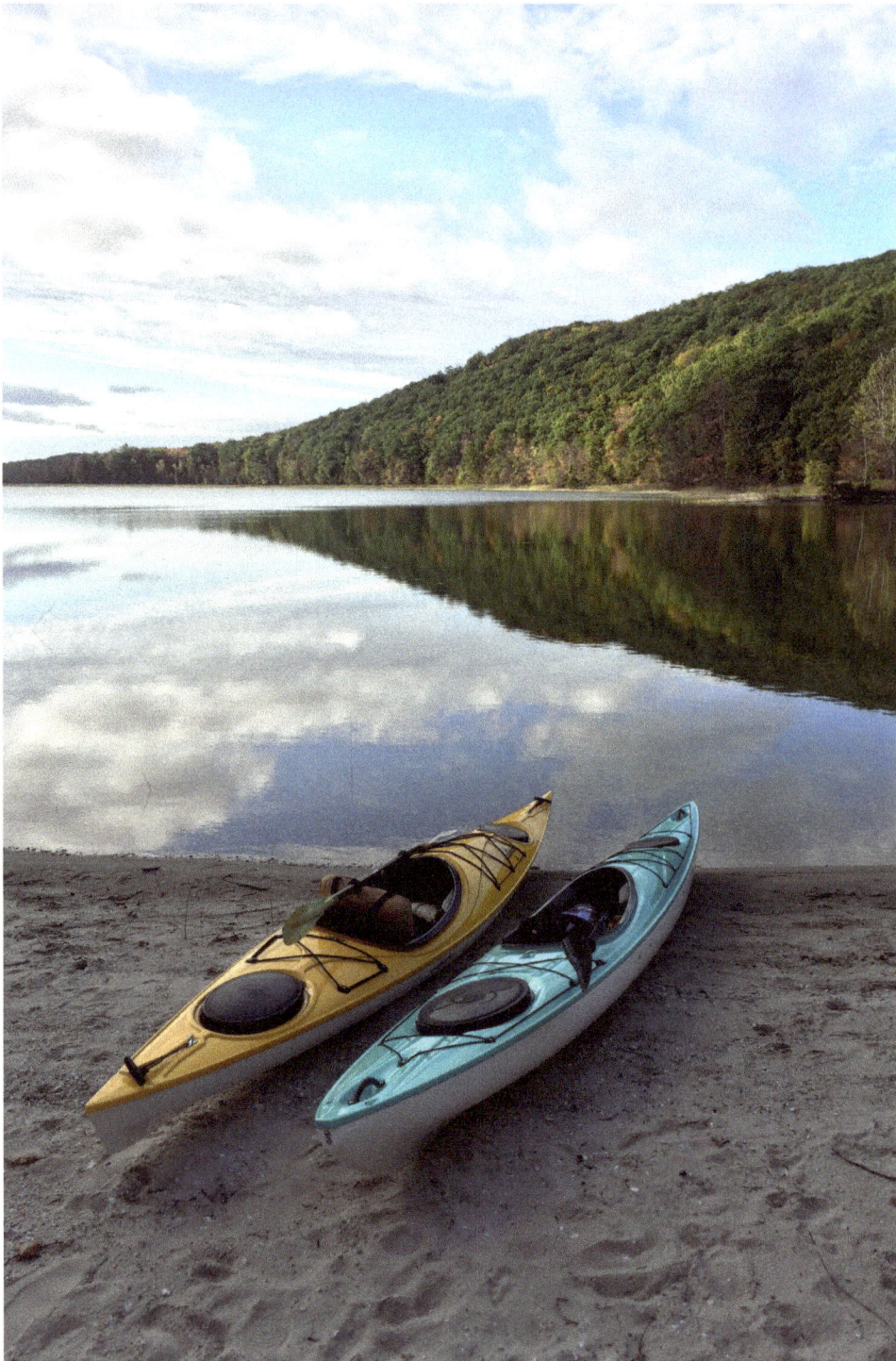

44

40 17 19

Shoal

12

142

17 21

17 25

18

15

21 17

27

21

112

21

24

10

Good
Harbor
Bay

Point

6

56

Shell
Lake

12

12

7

7

National

Narada
Lake

Lake Michigan

Lakeshore

22

Bass Lake

44°55'

2

5 4

6

School Lake

669

PLATE 5

BASS LAKE

This oval-shaped lake is a great choice for a quiet and leisurely paddle. There is a large, forested ridge to the west that makes for an interesting setting — especially in the fall when the trees are at peak color. Other than a cabin at the northeast corner, there are no homes or cottages — the perfect place to get away from things.

LOCATION: Bass Lake is located immediately south of M-22 and northeast of Glen Arbor. It's less than a mile from Bohemian Road (County Road 669), and just east of Little Traverse Lake.

ACCESS: There is a carry-in site off of M-22, near the northwest corner of the lake. You will have to park on the shoulder of M-22. A short path leads to Bass Lake's sandy shores. There are no amenities.

INFORMATION:

» This lake is about the same size as Shell Lake (around 90 acres). There is a 1.6 mile shoreline. Bass Lake is shallow, with no spot more than 10 feet deep.

» There is a short, man-made channel connecting Bass Lake with School Lake next door, to the south. There are no outlets.

COMMENTS:

» This is a quiet lake, even with M-22 right next door. In fact, a paddle on this little lake gives you an idea of what other, busier lakes were like before development and tourism. There is no development here — just a wooded shoreline and a place for you to listen to nature and the sound of your paddle against the water.

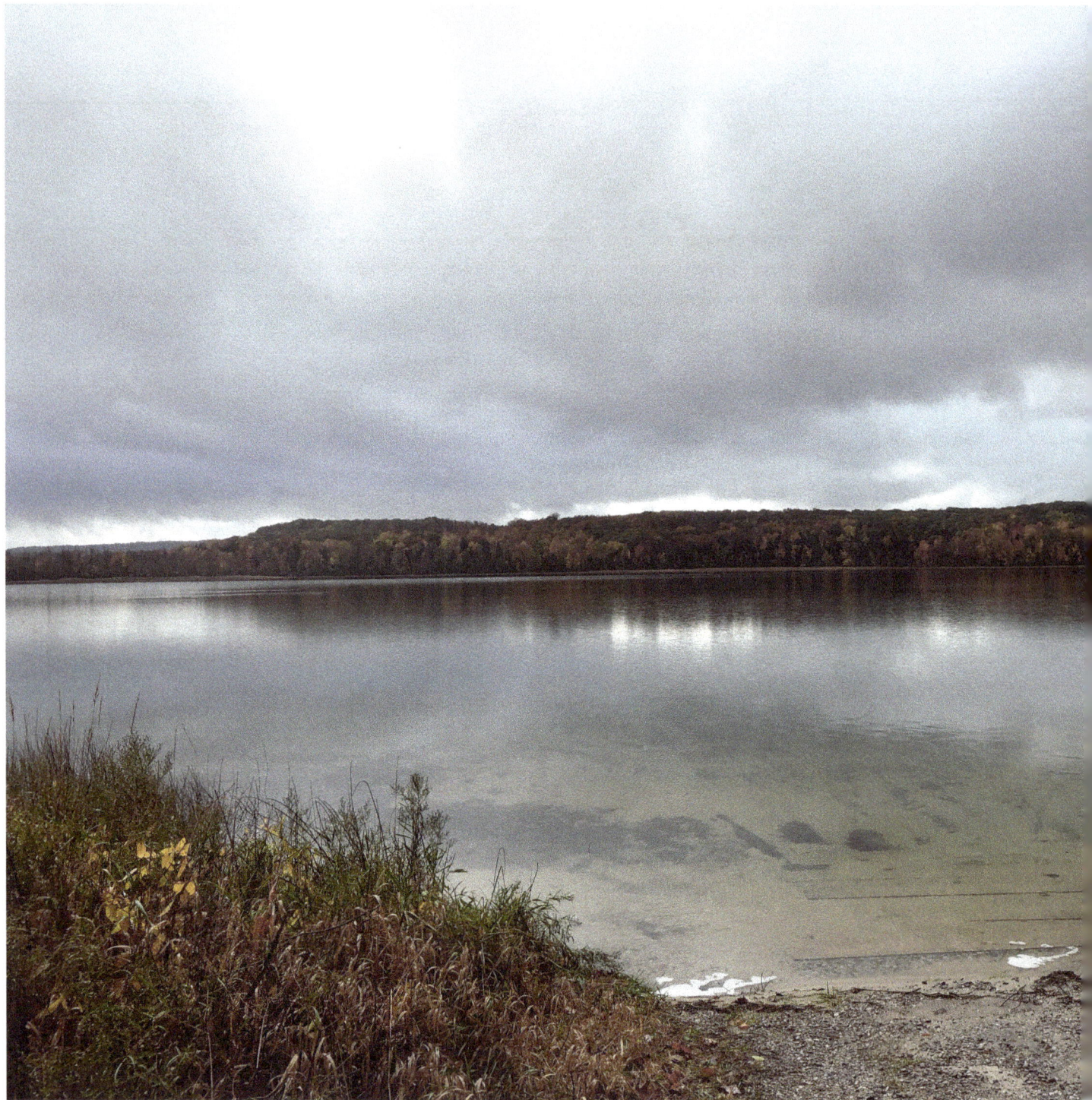

SCHOOL LAKE

School Lake, part of Sleeping Bear Dunes National Lakeshore, is a rounder, larger twin to Bass Lake to its north. Entirely undeveloped along its shoreline, the lake is surrounded by hills.

LOCATION: School Lake is immediately south of Bass Lake and east of Little Traverse Lake. It is 22 miles northwest of Traverse City.

ACCESS: There is an excellent concrete landing complete with parking and bathroom facilities located off of Bohemian Road (County Road 669), just south of the intersection of M-22. A National Park Pass is required at the site.

INFORMATION:

» This oval lake is 175 acres with a shoreline of 2.2 miles.

» Much of School Lake is quite shallow and sandy-bottomed. The middle of the lake averages 6 feet in depth. There is a much deeper area of the lake in a small appendage that juts out at the southwestern end of the lake. Depths in that little section of the lake reach 18 feet.

» Although the DNR map showed no inlets, there appeared to be a small tributary at the southern end. The same DNR map shows an intermittent, man-made outlet at the north end that connects School Lake with Bass Lake. When we paddled the lake, we explored that area on foot as it was dry at the time.

COMMENTS:

» School Lake can be kayaked as part of a package tour with nearby Bass and Shell Lakes. The experience of three, quiet lakes in such beautiful natural settings makes for a great day. We saw many migrating ducks and geese, and also saw lots of bass, perch, bluegill and minnows.

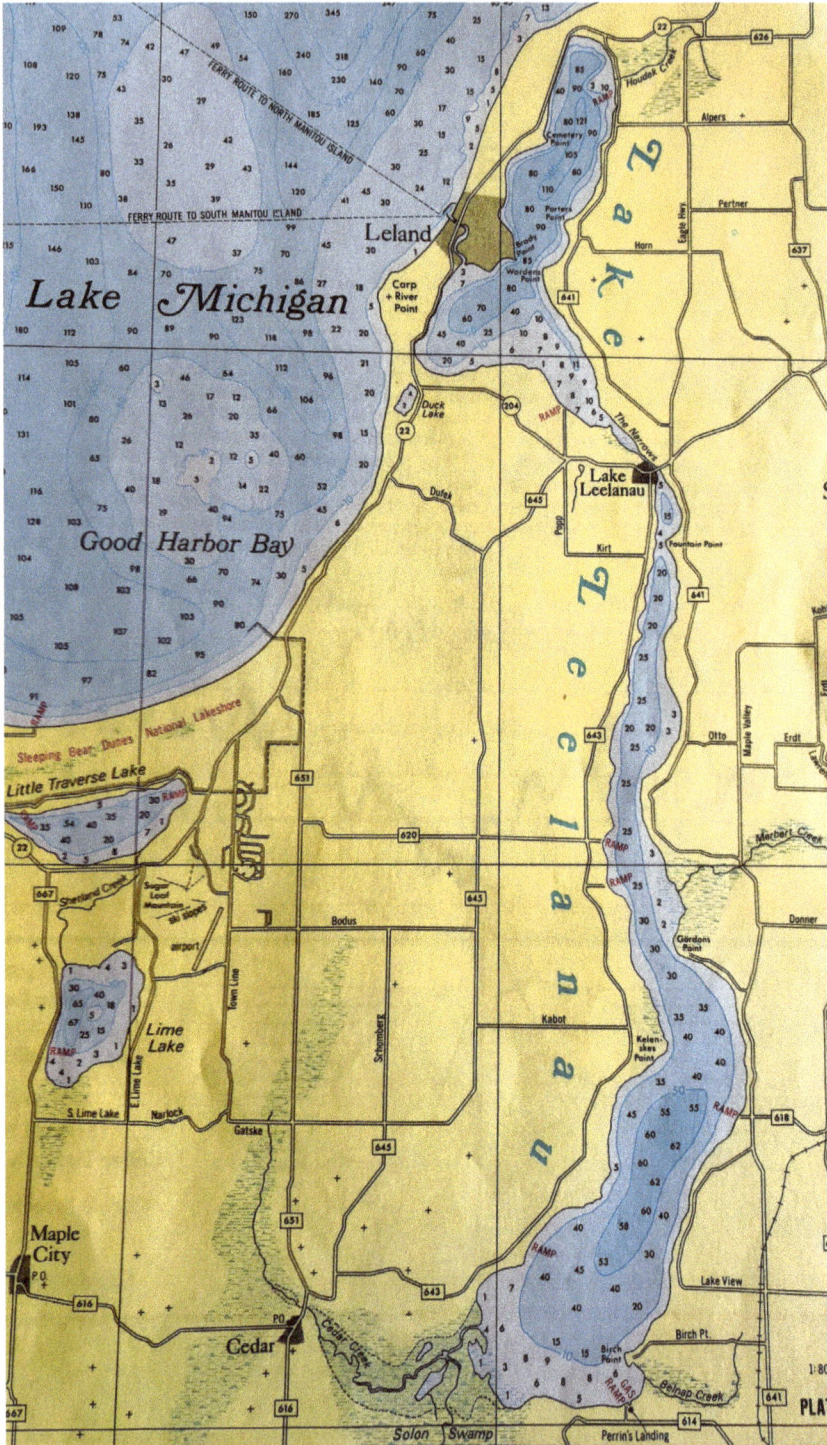

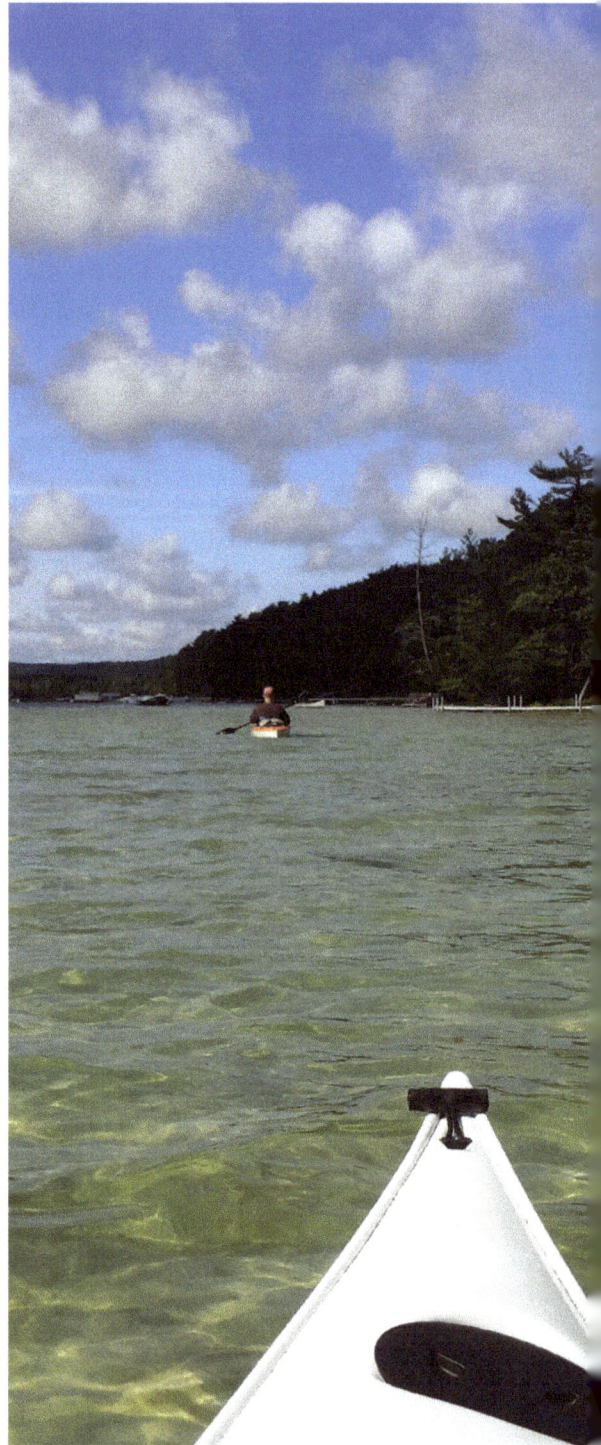

Lake Michigan

Good Harbor Bay

Leland

Corp + River Point

Duck Lake

Dufek

Sleeping Bear Dunes National Lakeshore

Little Traverse Lake

Lime Lake

S. Lime Lake   Narlock

Gatske

Maple City

Cedar

Solon Swamp   Perrin's Landing

Houdak Creek

Alpers

Partner

Horn

Lake

Lake Leelanau

The Narrows

Kirt

Fountain Point

Otto   Erdt

Machon Creek

Donner

Gordons Point

Kabot

Kelen-skes Point

Lake View

Birch Point   Birch Pt.

Belnap Creek

FERRY ROUTE TO NORTH MANITOU ISLAND

FERRY ROUTE TO SOUTH MANITOU ISLAND

Leelanau

Shetland Creek

Sugar Loaf Mountain ski slopes

airport

Town Line

E. Lime Lake

Schomberg

Bodus

Cedar Creek

PLAT

LITTLE TRAVERSE LAKE

Little Traverse Lake is a great, medium-sized, multi-sports lake located just south of Good Harbor Bay. The forests north of the lake are protected, as they are part of the Sleeping Bear Dunes National Lakeshore, but there are still lots of homes and cottages. Little Traverse Lake is a great alternative to the Big Lake when weather conditions are risky.

LOCATION: Little Traverse Lake is north of Maple City and Lime Lake, east of Bass and School Lakes and southwest of Leland.

ACCESS: We used two different Little Traverse Lake access sites on our different trips.

- Cleveland Township Park: This is the more improved of the two sites. It's on the north side of the lake, on Traverse Lake Road. The park has a concrete launch, a dock, parking, restrooms and a covered picnic pavilion.
- East end carry-in site: There's a sandy launch on the shore of Little Traverse Lake, 0.2 miles from M-22 on Traverse Lake Road. This spot has limited parking on the road and no dock or restrooms.

INFORMATION:

> » This lake is 640 acres and has a coastline of 5.0 miles.
> » Much of Little Traverse Lake is between 20 and 40 feet deep, with a 54-foot hole just east of the main boat launch.
> » Little Traverse Lake's main inlet is Shetland Creek. This creek flows a few miles south from Lime Lake, travels under M-22, then into Little Traverse Lake at its southeast side. The DNR map shows 24 small tributaries, mostly springs, entering the lake along its southern shoreline. The lake's only outlet is Shalda Creek, which flows out its western end and winds its way to Lake Michigan at Good Harbor Bay.

COMMENTS:

> » The views to the south, where Sugarloaf Mountain is a dominant feature, are a highlight of this lake. Sugarloaf Mountain Resorts was once the largest private employer in Leelanau County. Unfortunately, bad times and financial troubles closed the resort and it has been sitting vacant for decades. There is talk of Sugarloaf making a comeback in the near future. That would be great!
> » Little Traverse Lake holds a special place in my heart as it was here that Larry and I paddled just a few days after my dad's passing in 2013. Don Constant was my father, my high school football coach, a Michigan history teacher and a role model for my life. I remember that Larry and I didn't talk much on that paddle, but we didn't have to as the serenity of the lake, the fall colors on the maple trees and the sounds of our paddles dipping into the calm water were soothing enough.

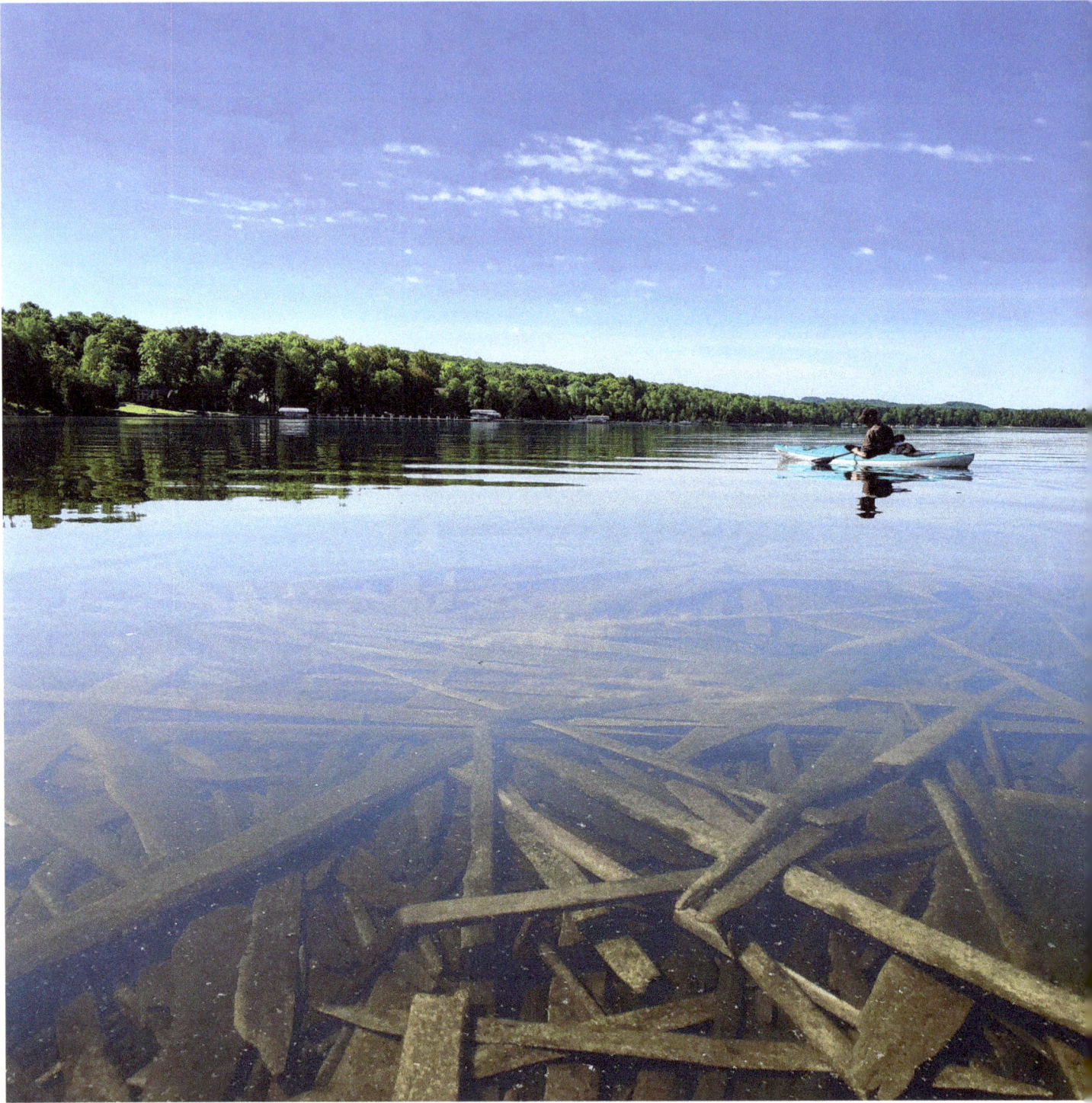

LIME LAKE

Lime Lake is well named, as it has the most beautiful green color. It's a medium-sized lake set between hills to the east and west, with flatter land to the north and south. Sugarloaf soars over this lake to the northeast.

LOCATION: Lime Lake is about 2 miles north of Maple City and just south of Little Traverse Lake and Good Harbor Bay.

ACCESS: We used the DNR boat launch on the southwest side of the lake, just off of Maple City Road (County Road 616). This site has a concrete launch, a dock, parking and bathroom facilities.

INFORMATION:

» Lime Lake is 670 acres (about the same size as Little Traverse Lake). Its shoreline is 5.0 miles long.

» Lime Lake has extended shallow areas, especially on its southern, eastern and northern shores, with a more extreme drop-off present on the western shore. Along the western side, there are areas reaching 67 feet deep. In the middle of the lake there is a shallow shoal only 5 feet deep — right next to the deepest part of the lake!

» The DNR map shows 11 inlets to Lime Lake, most of them small spring tributaries. There is a cedar swamp at the south end of the lake where Lime Creek is the main inlet.

» Shetland Creek flows out of Lime Lake at the northwest corner and eventually into Little Traverse Lake to the north.

COMMENTS:

» Teichner Preserve is at the northeast corner of the lake. These 40 acres include 200 feet of shoreline, wetlands and mature cedar trees. The preserve was donated by Martha Teichner, a *CBS Sunday Morning* personality, and it's named for her parents.

» On our paddle we saw large deposits of lumber — wood slabs and panels — on the bottom of the north end of the lake, remnants of a lumber mill long gone.

» Maple City is less than two miles south of Lime Lake. It was settled in 1866 when a shoe peg factory was built near several hundred acres of maple trees. The community was first called Peg Town, and then Maple. The post office named it Maple City. Today a great place in Maple City to get a bite to eat is Pegtown Station.

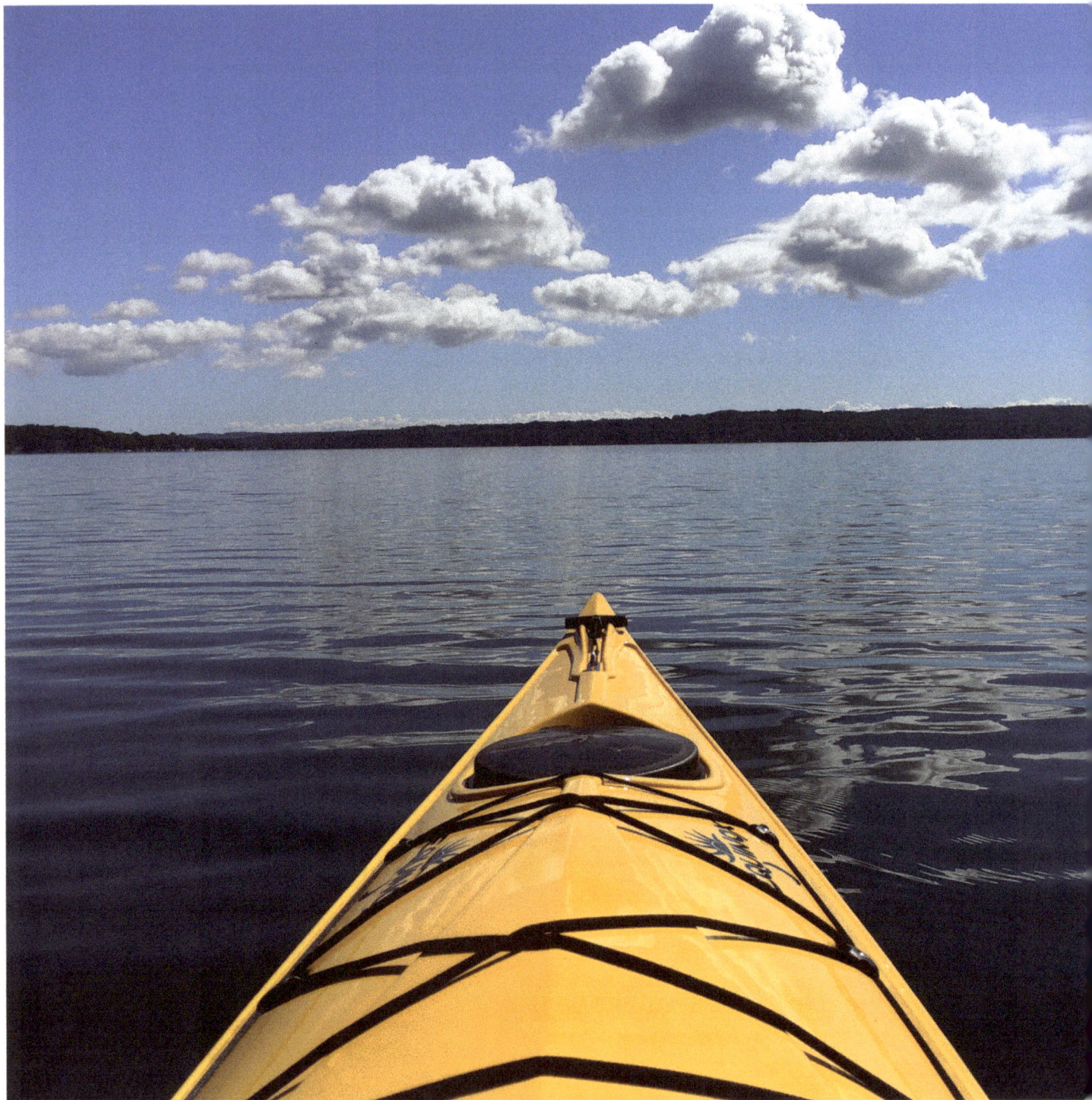

LAKE LEELANAU

This huge lake almost splits Leelanau County into two halves, and because of its central location, is often described as the "heart of Leelanau." Lake Leelanau is a grand lake, measuring 16 miles in length with a shoreline that comes in at 40 miles. We have paddled all of it! For the purposes of this book, Lake Leelanau is divided into two sections: North and South Lake Leelanau. Most locals do the same thing when describing the lake.

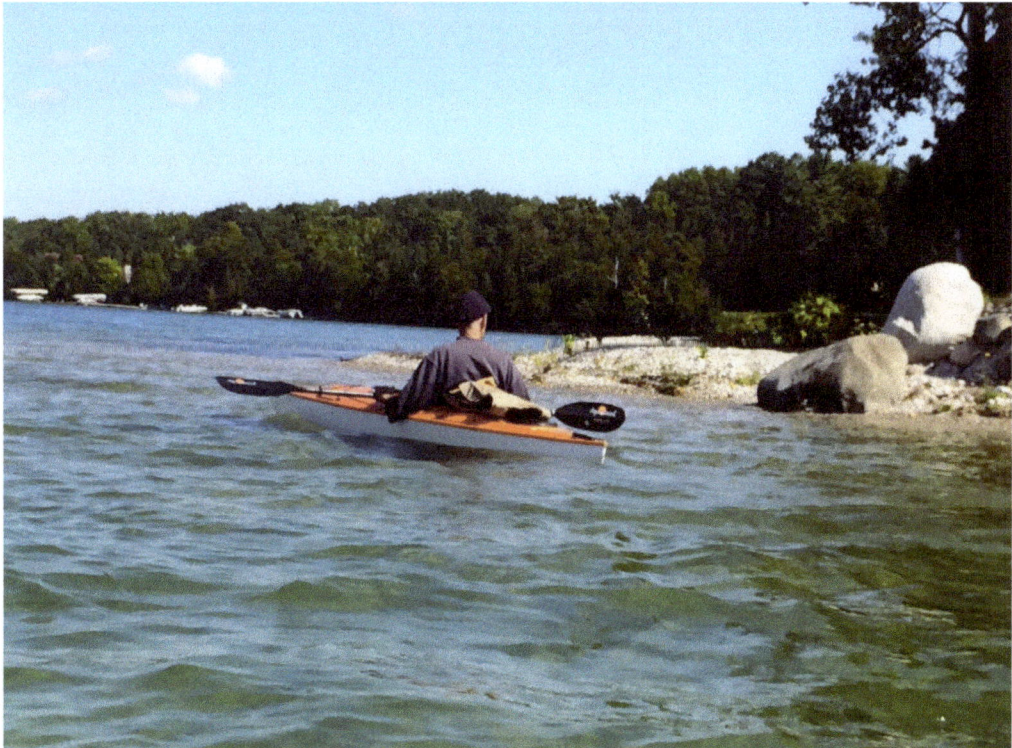

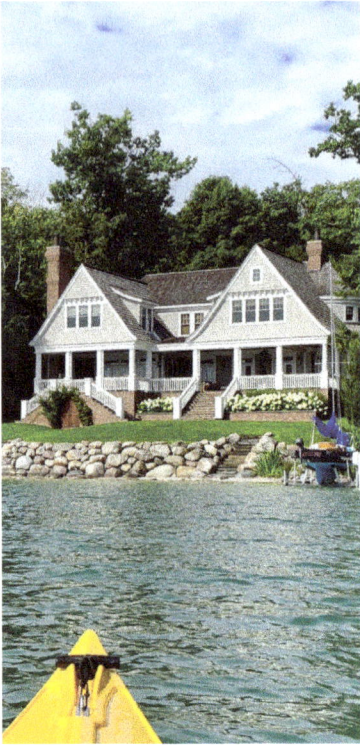

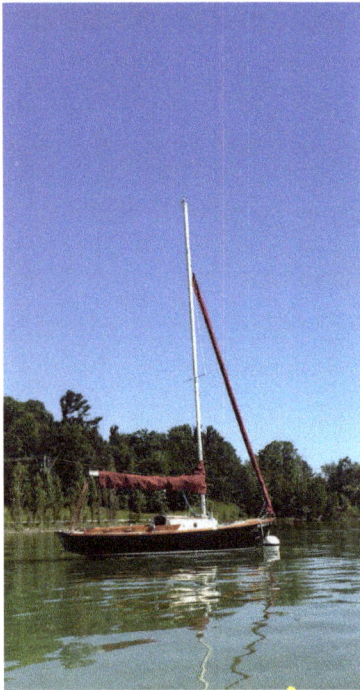

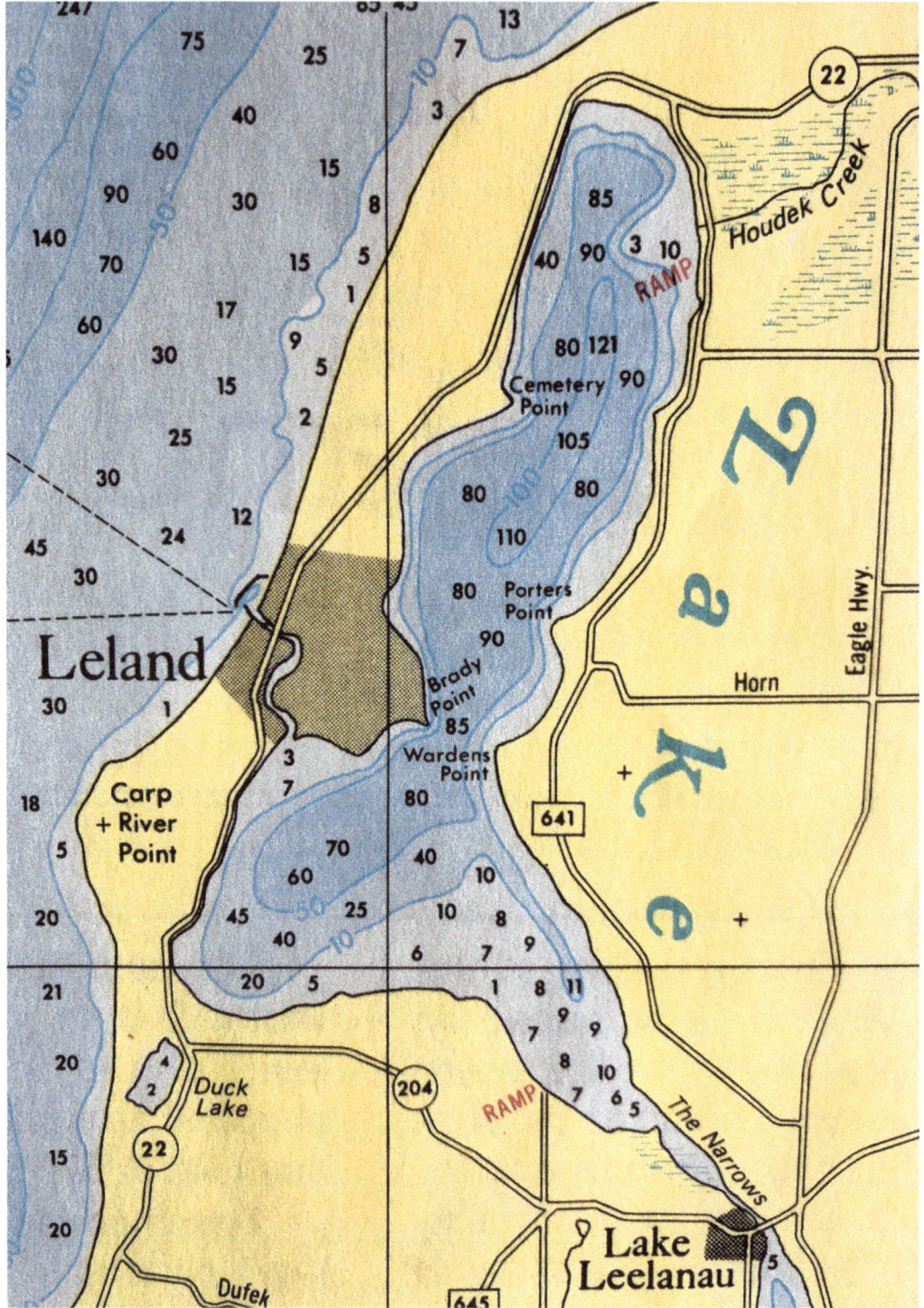

22

247

75

25

85 45

13

40

7

60

25

3

90

15

140

30

8

Houdek Creek

70

15

5

85

60

17

15

1

40

90

3 10

30

9

RAMP

15

5

80 121

25

2

Cemetery
Point

90

30

105

30

24

12

80

80

45

110

30

Porters
Point

80

Leland

90

30

1

Brady
Point

85

3

Wardens
Point

7

18

80

Carp
+ River
Point

5

70

40

20

60

10

45

40

10

8

40

6

7

9

21

20

5

1

8

11

9

9

20

4

7

8

10

2

Duck
Lake

8

7

6

5

22

204

RAMP

10

6 5

15

The Narrows

20

Lake
Leelanau

5

Dufek

645

641

Eagle Hwy.

Horn

Lake

NORTH LAKE LEELANAU

North Lake Leelanau is a large lake and, therefore, more vulnerable to winds, so care must be given to weather conditions. The lake has deep water so clear that its colors are often Caribbean-like. There are many amazing homes and cottages here, but there are also areas that are very natural. North Lake Leelanau is a great place for your next day trip.

LOCATION: North Lake Leelanau is found in the middle of Leelanau County, just east of Leland and north of the village of Lake Leelanau. M-22 passes by on its western and northern sides.

ACCESS: We have accessed North Lake Leelanau from several sites.

- The site closest to the village of Lake Leelanau is the park at the end of Popp Road, just a mile west of town. This site gives good access to the southern arm of North Lake Leelanau. There is no ramp, but there is a dock, picnic facilities, Porta Potties and parking.

- We have also used both DNR launches on the Leland River in Leland. One is located on River Street, next to the Bluebird Inn. The other is at the dead-end of Chandler Street. There is a concrete launch at the River Street access with limited parking. The Chandler Street launch has no ramp and is carry-in and out. Parking is off the street and limited.

- Another site we've used is Bartholomew Park in Leland, at the end of Pearl Street. This is a public beach and picnic area and a fine way to get on the North arm of North Lake Leelanau. Parking is available.

- The only other site we've used is the DNR access site at the extreme northeast side of the lake on North Lake Leelanau Drive (County Road 641), about a half mile south of M-22. This site includes a concrete launch, a small picnic area, Porta Potties and parking.

INFORMATION:

- » North Lake Leelanau is 2,950 acres. (Only South Lake Leelanau and Big Glen Lake are bigger.) It has a shoreline of 14.9 miles.

- » The maximum depth is 121 feet — you can find that in the middle of the north arm, north of Cemetery Point. The average is closer to 90 feet. As you get closer to The Narrows, the lake averages 8 feet.

- » The main inlet to North Lake Leelanau is The Narrows that connect North and South Leelanau.

- » The other main inlet is Houdek Creek, on its far northeast section, north of Alpers Road.

- » The DNR map shows 7 smaller tributaries entering North Lake Leelanau, mainly along its southern and eastern shores.

- » This lake's only outlet is the Leland River, which flows through Leland and Fishtown and on into Lake Michigan.

COMMENTS:

- » The shape of North Lake Leelanau allows the paddler the option of touring the north arm and the south arm on separate day trips. We put in at the DNR site at the northeast corner of the north arm, and toured the lake counterclockwise to Brady's Point. We then cut across to Warden's Point and continued north back to our vehicle. This took us about 3 hours in near-perfect conditions.

- » I think this is one of the most beautiful paddles of all Leelanau lakes. The water is particularly pretty in this area and the shore is nicely wooded. The estates, homes and cottages are interesting to view from the water. Most of these homes can't be seen from M-22 or County Road 641, but they are in plain view from a kayak.

- » We paddled around the south arm in the summer of 2017. We put in at the Popp Road access site, west of the village of Lake Leelanau, and traversed the lake clockwise, along with a short paddle up and back on the Leland River. We crossed from Brady Point to Warden's Point, paddled to The Narrows and then back to Popp Road. This took us about 3 hours, again in near perfect conditions. The clarity of the water and the unlimited visibility made for a spectacular day. What I remember from that day were the puffy clouds that made for great pics as we crossed the lake.

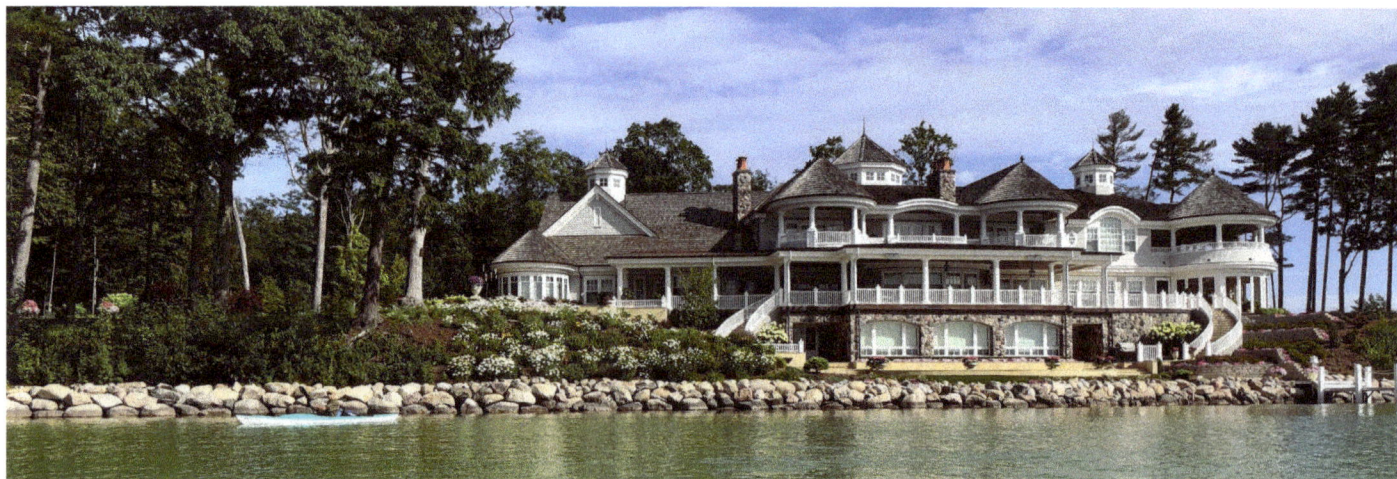

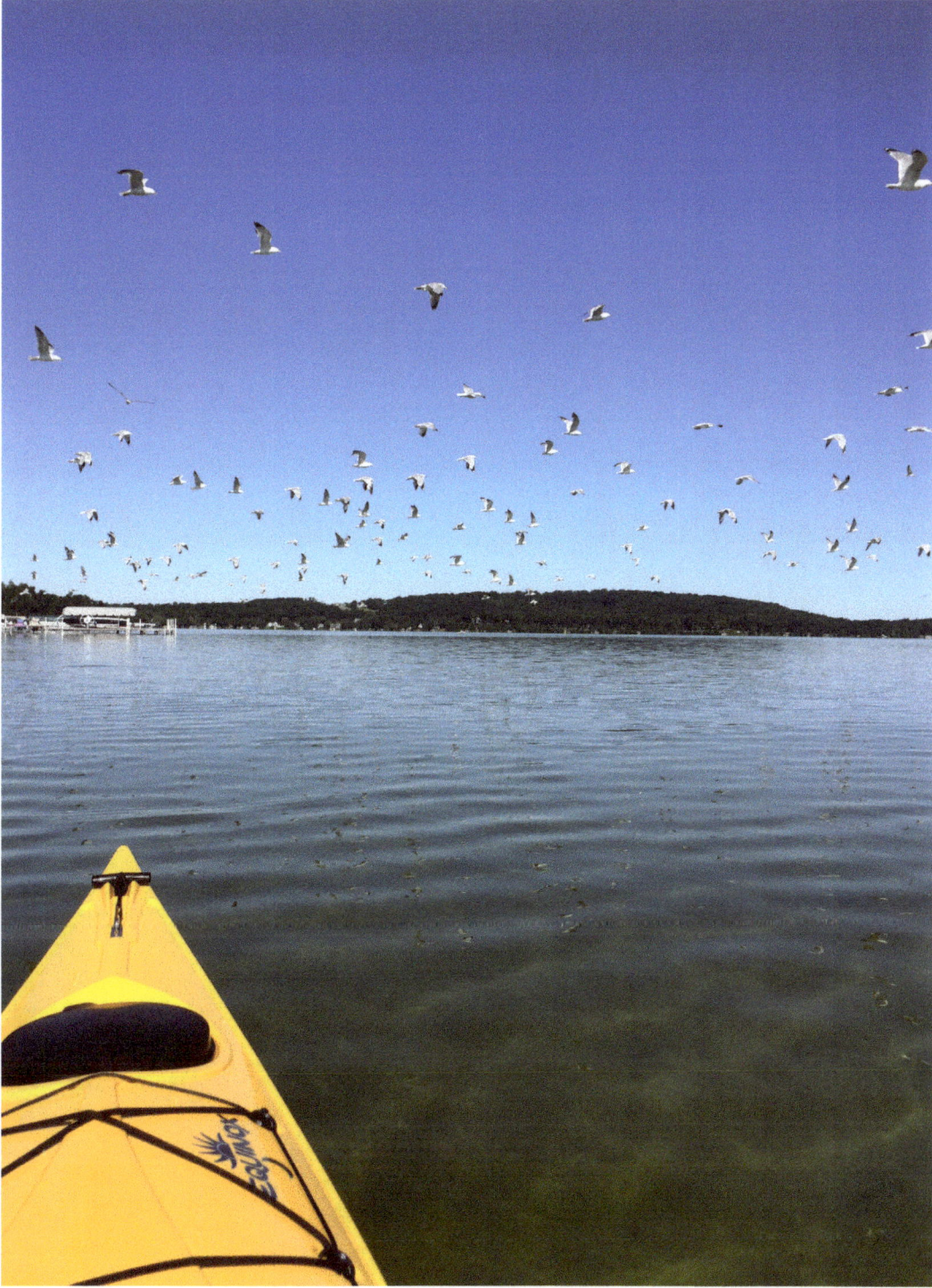

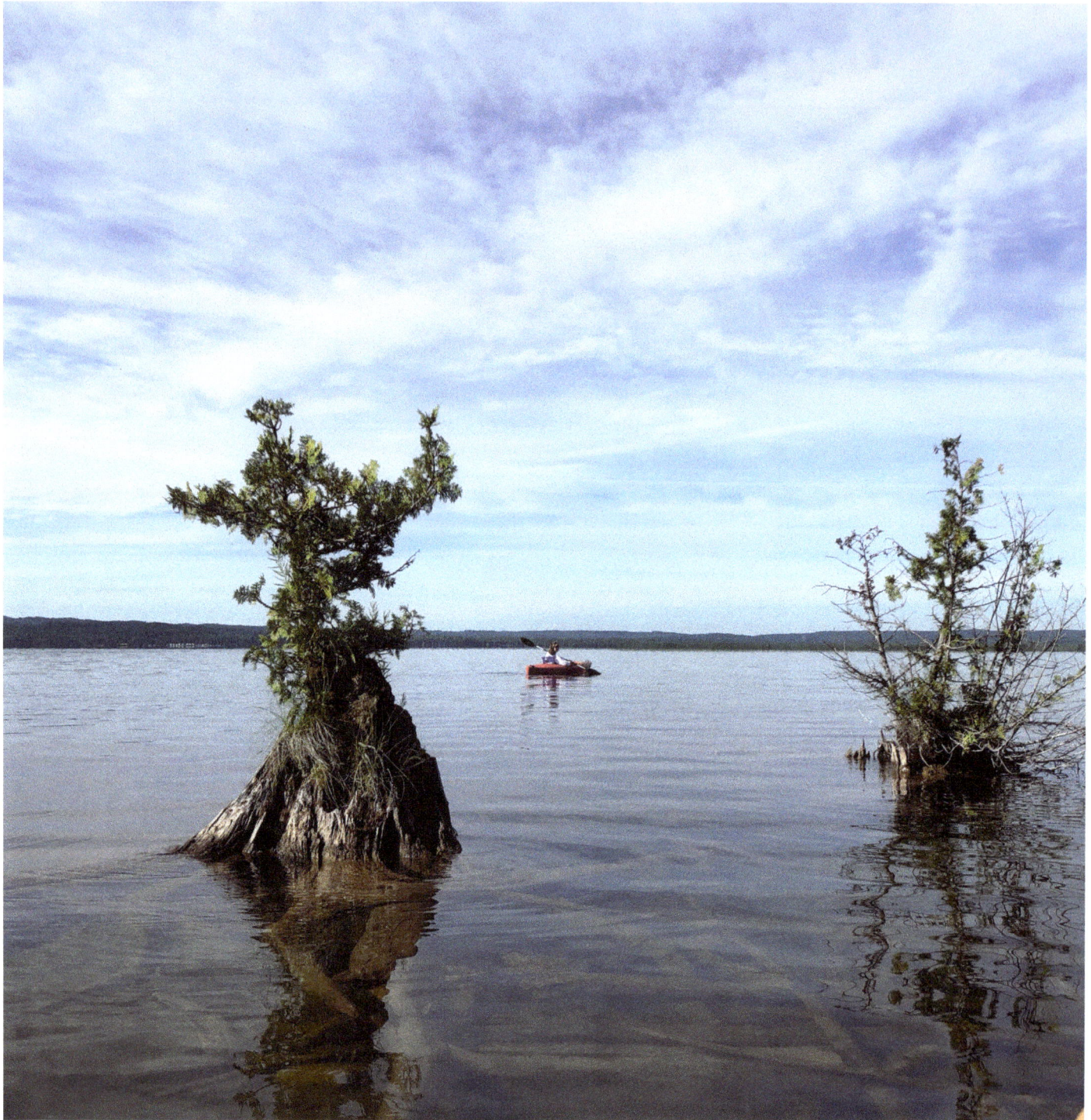

SOUTH LAKE LEELANAU

This part of Lake Leelanau has a different look and feel than North Lake Leelanau. At the north end it is elongated and quite shallow. At the southern end it is much wider and deeper. Be aware that the surrounding hills and the open waters of the lake can create quite a wind tunnel effect. Southwest winds can be particularly tricky.

LOCATION: South Lake Leelanau runs through the south central part of Leelanau County. It is south of the village of Lake Leelanau and The Narrows, east of Cedar and northwest of Traverse City.

ACCESS: This lake has many access points. Here are the ones we have visited or used:

- The access site closest to Traverse City is the landing on the extreme south end of the lake at Perrin's Landing on Fouch Road (County Road 614). There is limited parking on the road, a small dock and no restrooms.

- Midway up the eastern shore of South Lake Leelanau is the Bingham Landing DNR launch site. This site is at the intersection of Bingham Road and Lake Leelanau Drive (County Road 641). Here there is a concrete landing, a dock, plenty of parking and a restroom.

- Closer to The Narrows and the village of Lake Leelanau, there is another DNR launch on the eastern shore, less than 0.1 mile from the intersection of M-204 and South Lake Leelanau Drive. There is plenty of parking, a concrete launch, a dock and restroom facilities.

- I have visited and used two separate western launches on the northerly, mid-portions of this long lake. The most northerly is a ramp at the intersection of Lakeshore Drive (County Road 643) and Hohnke Road (County Road 620). This site is part of Centerville Park. It has a launch, a dock, parking and restroom facilities. A second launch is nearby, to the south. There is a DNR access site on Lakeshore Drive (County Road 643), about a mile north of Kabot Road. This site has a concrete launch, a dock, a gravel parking area and a restroom.

- The Solon Township Park offers a launch site that is closer to the south end of the lake. The launch is about 3 miles from Cedar, and can be reached by taking County Road 651 north out of Cedar, turning right on Schomberg Road (County Road 645), then taking another quick right on Lakeshore Drive (County Road 643) to Solon Park Road. This site has a small concrete launch, a dock, some parking and a restroom.

- If you don't mind the 3.5-mile paddle to South Lake Leelanau, you can use the launch on the north side of the Cedar River right in Cedar. This site has a launch, a dock, plenty of parking, picnic facilities across the footbridge and Porta Potties.

INFORMATION:

» Lake Leelanau is by far the largest in the county, coming in at 5,693 acres with a whopping 26.2 mile shoreline. It took us several day trips to complete our journey around this huge lake.

» South Lake Leelanau has an average depth of just 25 feet, with the deepest areas (62 feet) found in the middle, off Lake View and Bingham roads. The northern, more narrow part of South Lake Leelanau has a channel that is consistently around 25 to 30 feet deep. North of Fountain Point, the depth decreases and there is a no wake zone for power boats.

» The village of Lake Leelanau is located where M-204 crosses the narrow's of Lake Leelanau. The Native Americans called the spot Ke-ski-bi-ag, which meant, "Narrow body of water." Simon and Jacob Schaub arrived at the narrows in 1855 and it was given the name Provemont, believed to be a shortened version of "improvement." In 1924, the US Post Office was renamed Lake Leelanau.

» There are over 20 inlets. The largest ones include:

  • Cedar River in the southwest Solon Swamp section of the lake.

  • Weisler Creek, west of Perrin's Landing in the southern section.

  • Mann Creek in the southern section.

  • Belnap Creek in the southeast corner between Perrin's Landing and Birch Point.

  • Merbert Creek in the east, midway up the lake past Gordon's Point.

  • Rice Creek on the west side of the lake, a few miles north of the Cedar River inlet.

» The only outlet for South Lake Leelanau is at The Narrows, near the extreme northern end of the lake. This is a no-wake zone for boaters and a great spot to see great blue herons, song sparrows and redwing blackbirds. Or take a break from paddling for a rest, a bite to eat and enjoy the boat traffic slowly passing by.

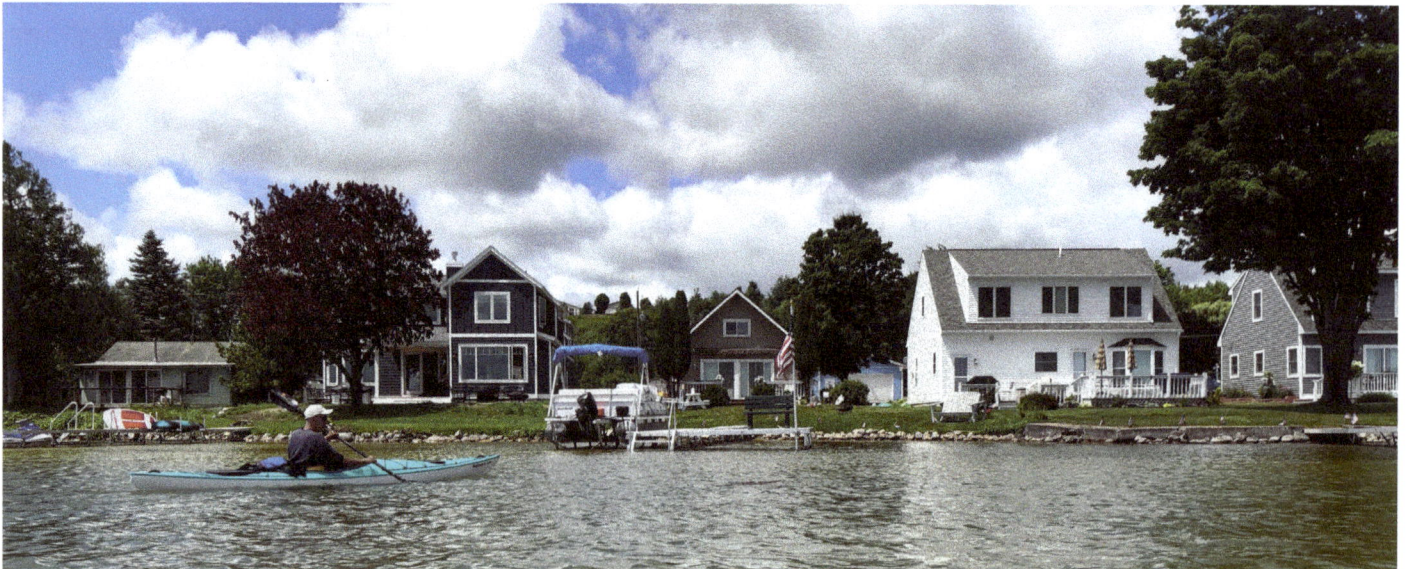

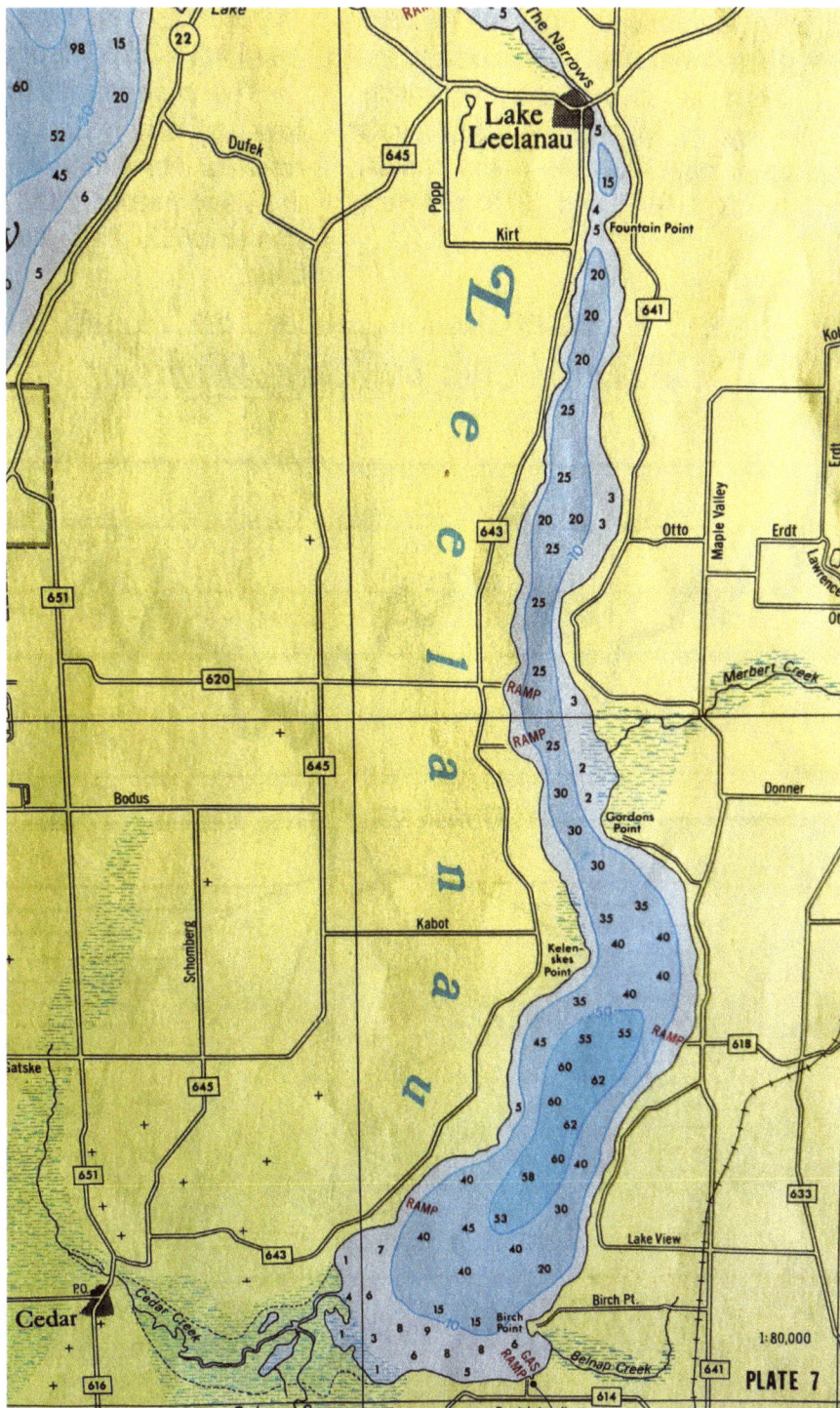

COMMENTS:

» Lake Leelanau lake levels are regulated by a dam in Leland. When the dam was built in 1854, the levels of both the north and south arms rose an amazing 12 feet. What was once 3 lakes linked by a river became a single lake. People, supplies and products for sale were transported by schooners and steamers up and down the lake.

» The remnants of lumber days long gone can still be seen in the massive logs, huge stumps and timbers on the bottom of the lake.

» Fountain Point is on the northeastern section of The Narrows, just south of the village of Lake Leelanau. Around 1860, one of the area's first settlers tried drilling for oil, and instead of an oil gusher, he hit a gusher of sparkling pure water at a depth of 900 feet. The land changed hands several times until, in 1889, a buyer from Cincinnati, Ohio, established The Fountain Point House, a Victorian-style resort for summer guests. The railroad from Traverse City ran by the location on its route to Northport and improved Fountain Point's accessibility. More and more cottages were built, and the resort became a popular summer destination. Today, Fountain Point is still run as a recreational hotel and resort, and hosts concerts and weddings. It is also home to the Lake Leelanau Rowing Club. Rowing teams from colleges use this quiet section of South Lake Leelanau for practices and contests.

» In the late 1800s, South Lake Leelanau had many small wooden steamships taking goods and tourists the length of the lake, from Perrin's Landing, on the far south end, to Leland, with many stops in between.

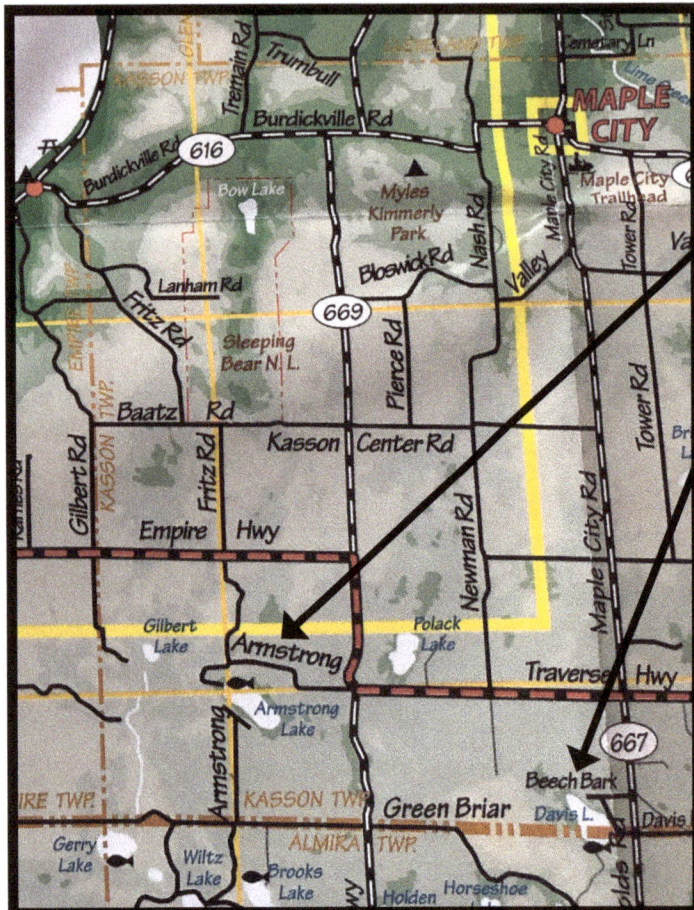

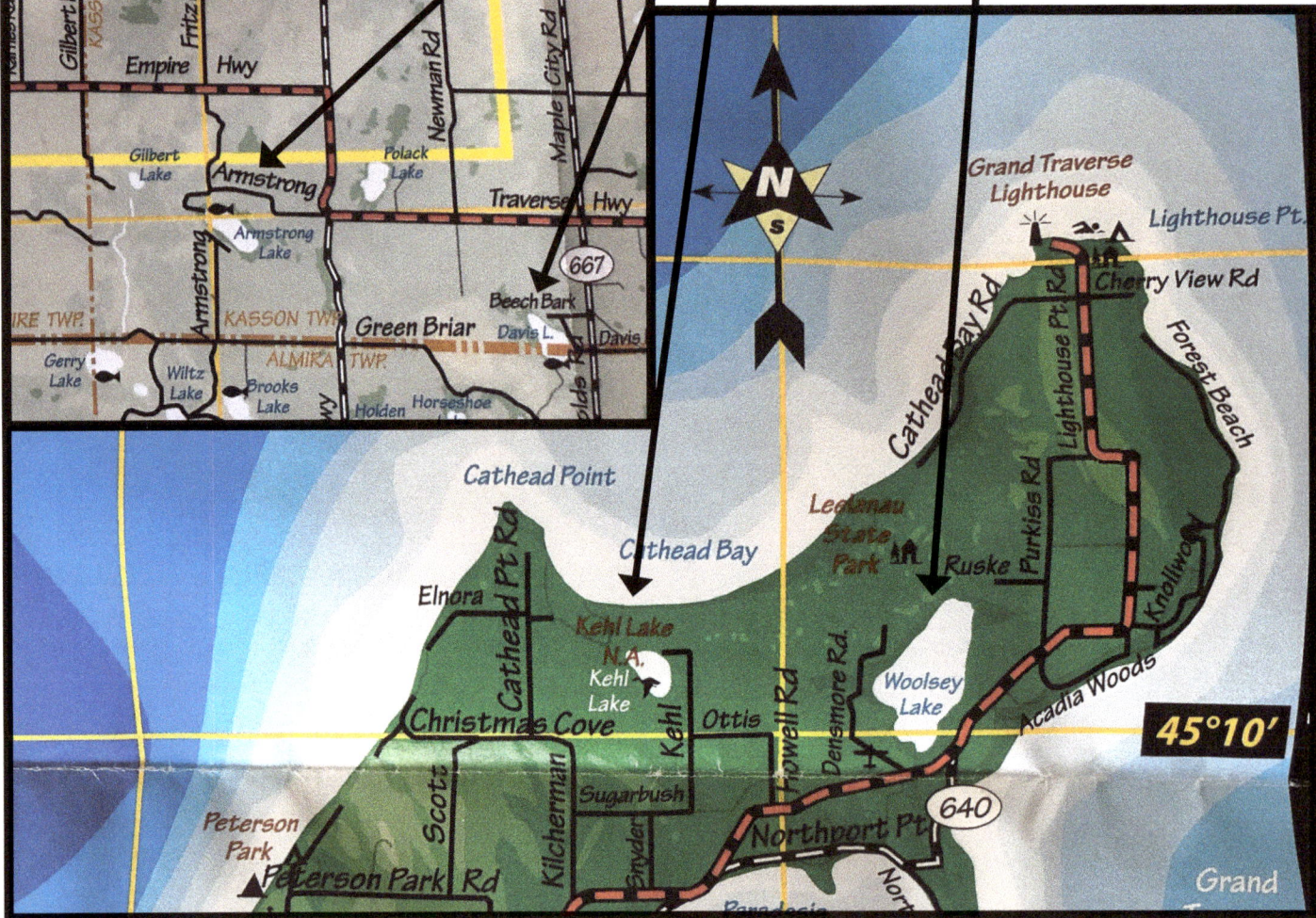

ARMSTRONG LAKE

DAVIS LAKE

KEHL LAKE

WOOLSEY LAKE

45°10'

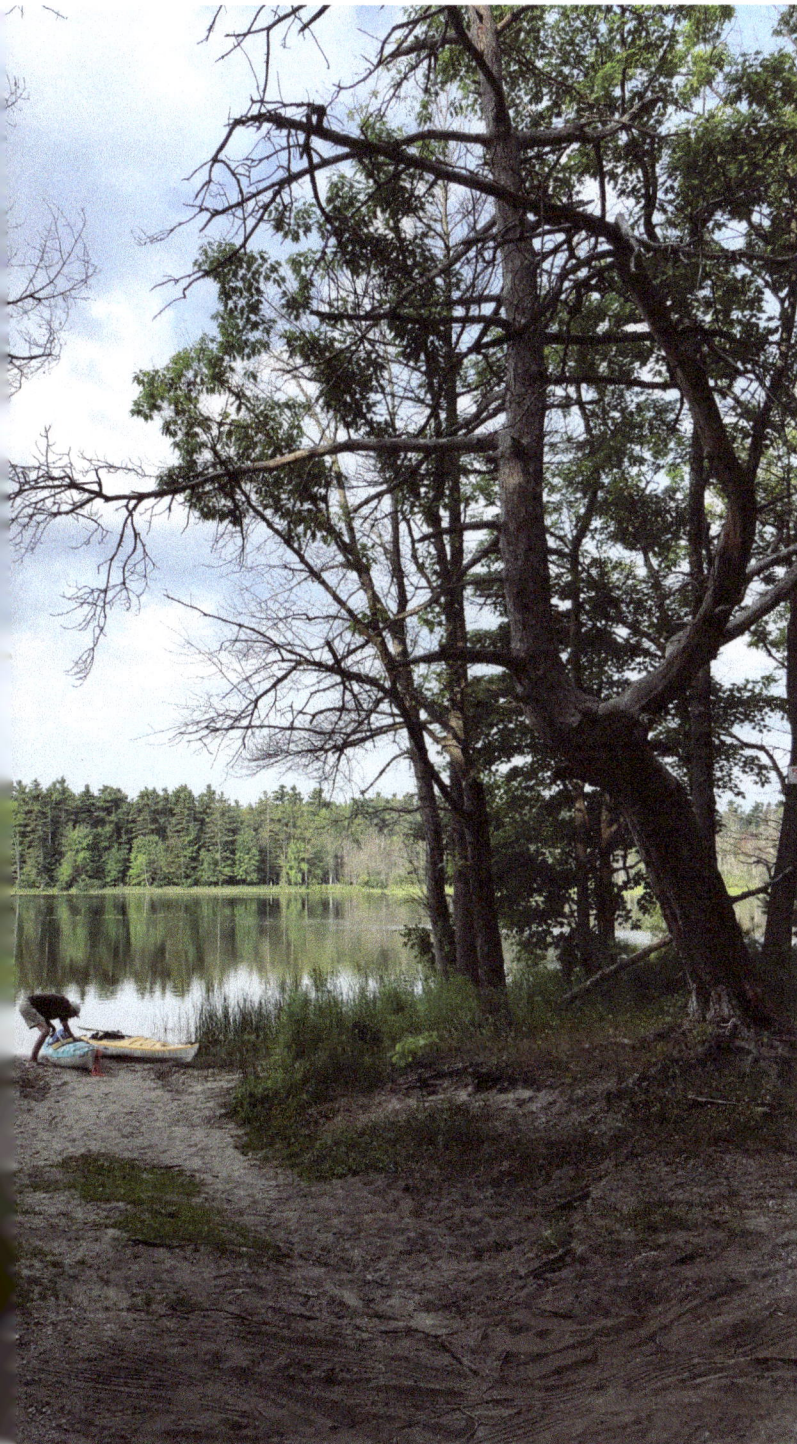

FOUR LITTLE LAKES:
TWO IN LEELANAU'S SOUTH AND TWO IN LEELANAU'S NORTH

Not all the lakes in Leelanau are well known. Davis Lake and Armstrong Lake are located south of M-72 on the extreme southern border of Leelanau. At the northern tip of Leelanau you will find Kehl Lake near the Grand Traverse Lighthouse and just to its east, Woolsey Lake, also called Mud Lake. Woolsey Lake proved too difficult for us to get to in late summer and low water tables. It will have to wait until the future when there is higher water, but it is included here for those who might want to explore it.

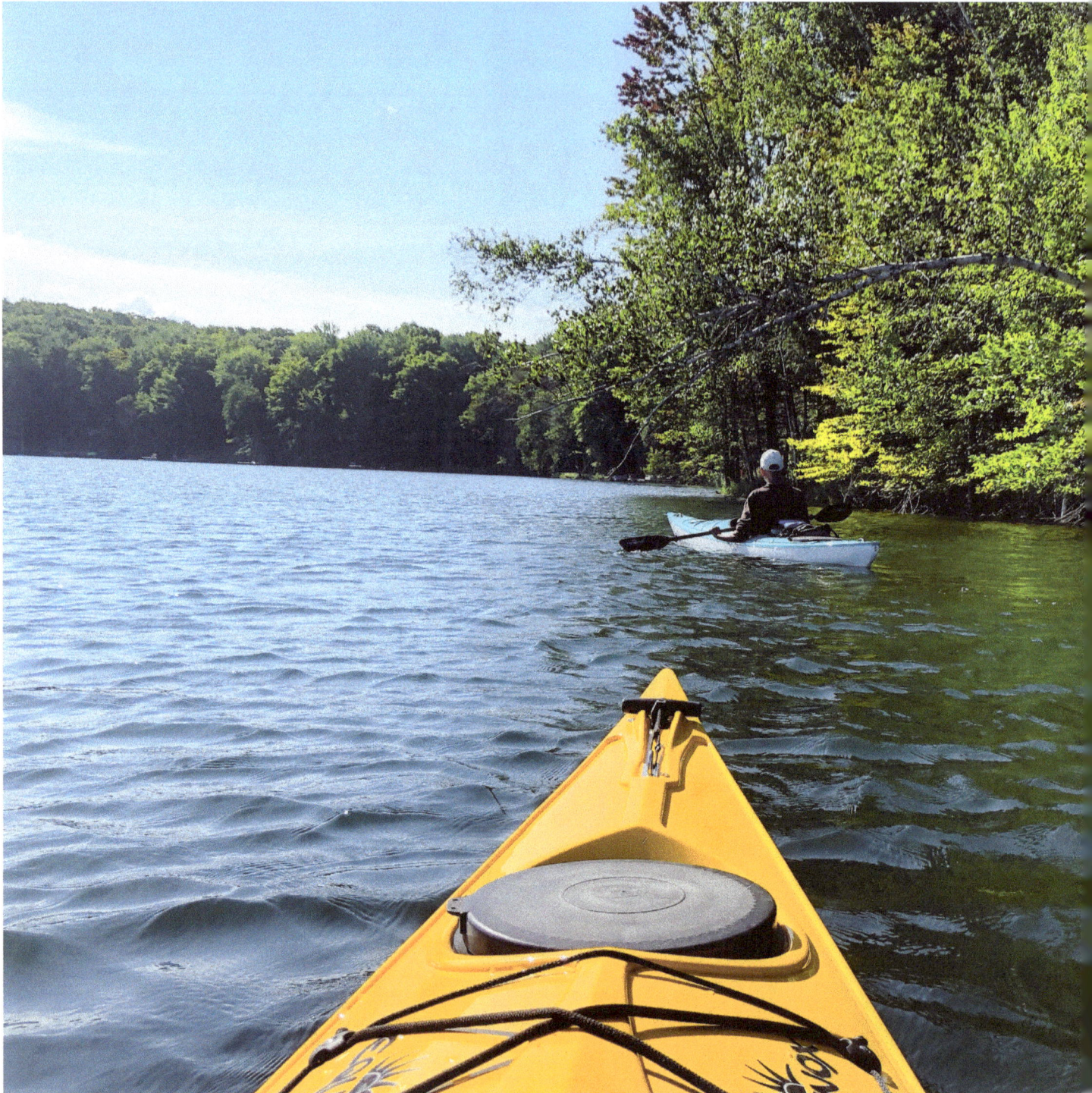

ARMSTRONG LAKE

We paddled the slightly larger Armstrong Lake on the same morning we visited Davis Lake. This is another hidden gem that is pretty easy to get to and enjoy—especially on a windy day. It took us less than 30 minutes to load up from our paddle on Davis Lake to being on the water on Armstrong Lake.

LOCATION: Armstrong Lake is located about 3 miles west of Davis Lake and about 11 miles west of Traverse City and 7 miles east of Empire. This little gem is just north of Benzie County's Pearl Lake and southeast of Big Glen Lake.

ACCESS: Look for Armstrong Road where M-72 makes a hard 90 degree turn to the north (right) as you travel from west from Traverse City. Take a left on Armstrong Road and go just less than a mile to the lake access road. Go another 0.3 miles to the gravel ramp. This is another DNR Access Site and has parking and a restroom available.

INFORMATION:

» Armstrong Lake has a slightly rectangular shape. It is definitely on the smaller size, coming in at 50 acres and a shoreline of 1.2 miles. It took us about 30 minutes to paddle Armstrong Lake at a leisurely pace.

» It had a decent depth of at least 10 feet or more.

» There are no inlets or outlets to Armstrong Lake that we could find.

COMMENTS:

» This lake has a very nice combination of woods and homes. There were some very nice houses and cottages to look at on Armstrong Lake. The lake is located near some small hills and ridges and would be a delightful place for a paddle in the fall to experience the beautiful Leelanau autumn colors.

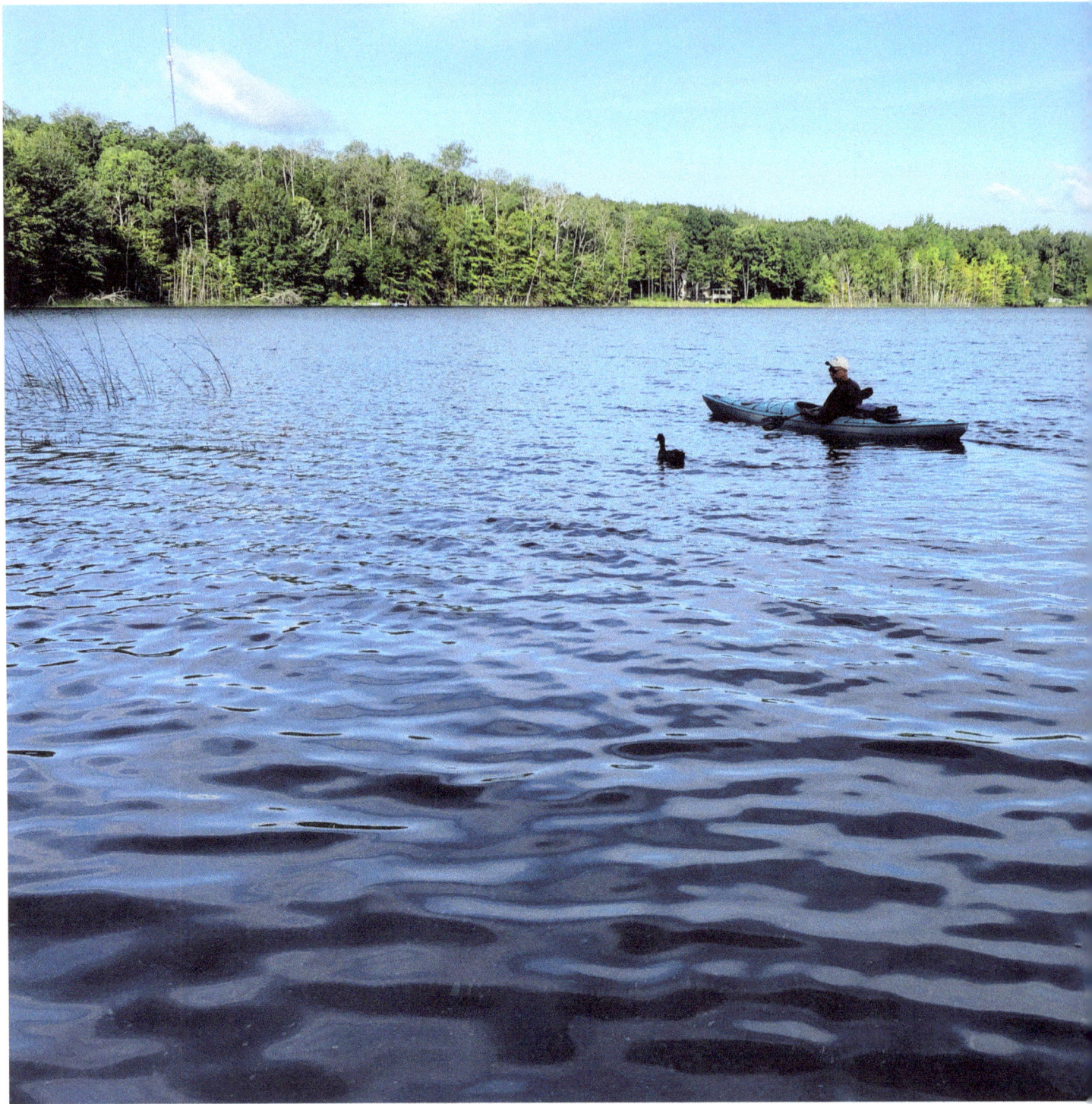

DAVIS LAKE

If you are looking for a quiet paddle on a quiet pretty lake that is off the beaten path, then Davis Lake is for you. This small beauty of a lake is a great option on a windy day as it sits inland from Lake Michigan and is surrounded by some low hills. The day we paddled Davis Lake we were escorted around much of the lake by the biggest and tamest Mallard Duck that I've ever seen. I think he either wanted to show us his paddling skills or maybe he just wanted a handout.

LOCATION: Davis Lake is located south of M-72 and about 8 miles west of Traverse City and about 10 miles east of Empire. This tear-dropped shape lake sits on the Leelanau/Benzie County line. (20% of the lake actually lies in Ben-zie County.)

ACCESS: Davis Lake is accessed off Davis Lake Road, south of M-72. At the intersection of M-72 and County Road 667, turn left on 667 (Reynolds Road). Go south about a mile to Davis Lake Road and turn right (west) and go less than ½ mile to the access road to the landing. This is a DNR access site and has a gravel launch, parking and a restroom.

INFORMATION:

» Davis Lake has 34 acres and a shoreline of 1.0 miles.

» Its deepest area is 40 feet, surprising for a lake of this size.

» Davis Lake has exceptionally clear water and is very wooded and scenic.

» The DNR map shows no inlets or outlets for Davis Lake.

COMMENTS:

» The morning we paddled Davis Lake there was very little activity on the lake or shoreline (other than that big duck). There are between 15 and 20 homes and cottages distributed around the shore. It was a gorgeous late August day with perfect conditions. It took us about 25 minutes to go around the perimeter of the lake.

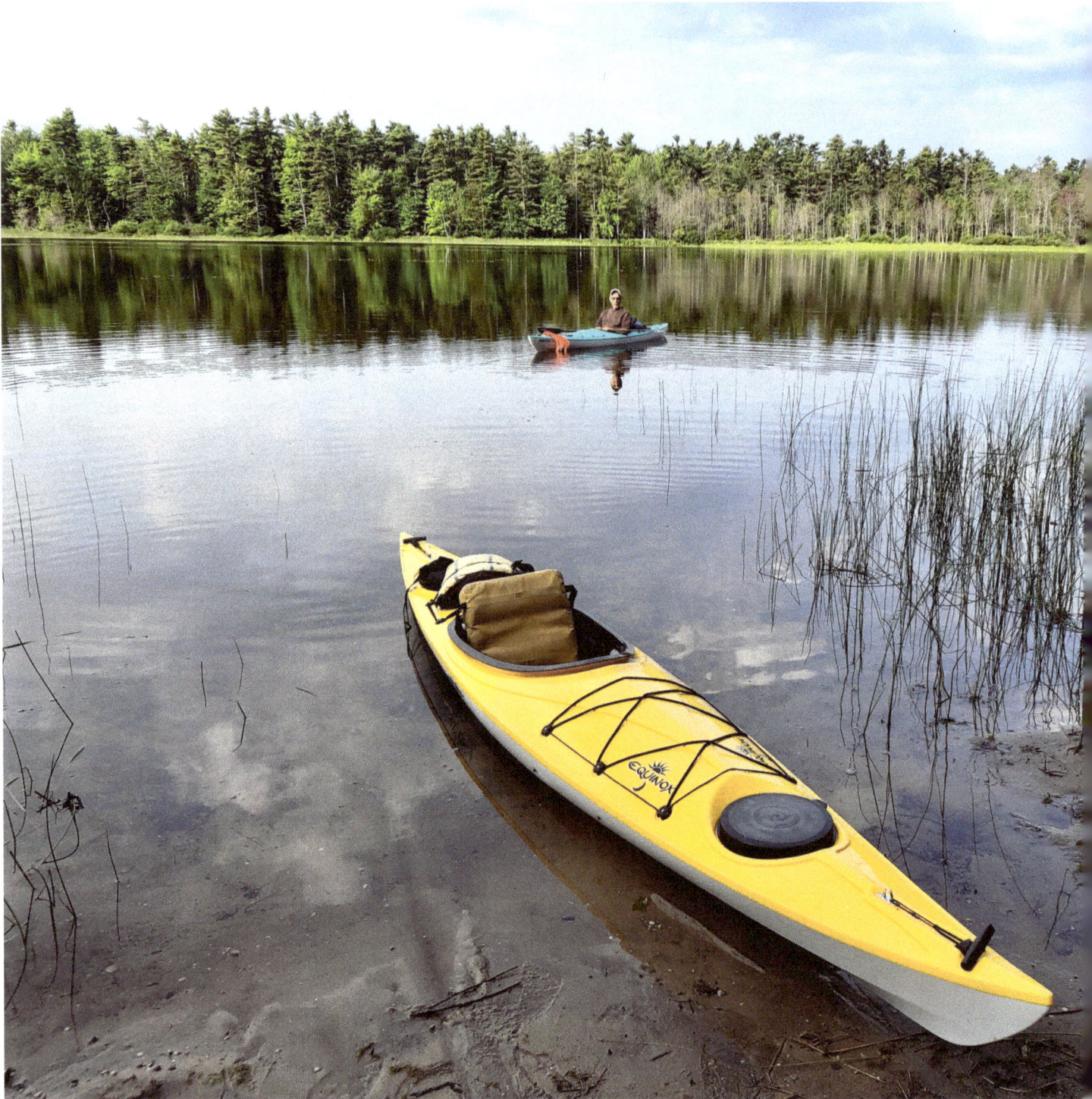

KEHL LAKE

We took a day trip to Kehl Lake on August 15, 2018.

Kehl Lake is located at the tip of Leelanau, roughly 30 miles north of Traverse City, close to Cathead Point. It is part of the Kehl Lake Natural Area and the Leelanau State Park. Kehl Lake has only a small amount of private land near the launch site. Most of the shoreline is wetlands or for-est. There is one house that can be seen from the water and it is located just south of the access site. The day we paddled Kehl Lake I believe we "surprised" a person on the deck of that house which made me think "visi-tors" on the lake aren't that common. Some locals refer to this lake as Leg Lake.

LOCATION: Kehl Lake is about 3 miles north of Northport, just west of Mud Lake, and about a quarter mile from Cathead Bay and Lake Michigan.

ACCESS: Kehl Lake is accessed from Kehl Road. To get to the access site, go north out of Northport on M-201 about 2 miles to Snyder Road. Turn left (north) on Snyder for a half mile to Sugarbush Road. Turn right (east) for 1 quarter mile where it ends at Kehl Road. Turn left (north) on Kehl and go about 1 mile to the launch site at Kehl Lake. The launch is fairly rustic with no restroom, limited parking and no dock.

INFORMATION:

» Kehl Lake has an area of 27 acres and a shoreline of 0.9 miles. It took us about 25 minutes to paddle the shoreline, with a small time to pause to watch a Loon at the southern end. Kehl Lake has a rounded triangle shape and there is a small bay located at the northwest corner that comes and goes depending on the water table.

» The deepest part of the lake is 20 feet and has one inlet near that small bay. There don't appear to be any outlets.

COMMENTS:

» Kehl Lake was one of the best surprises of any of our trips. I did not ex-pect such a pretty lake. The lake looks like it might be prime Bald Eagle and/or Osprey habitat. Kehl Lake is just the lake for a kayaker who wants to take in the quiet, natural beauty of Leelanau.

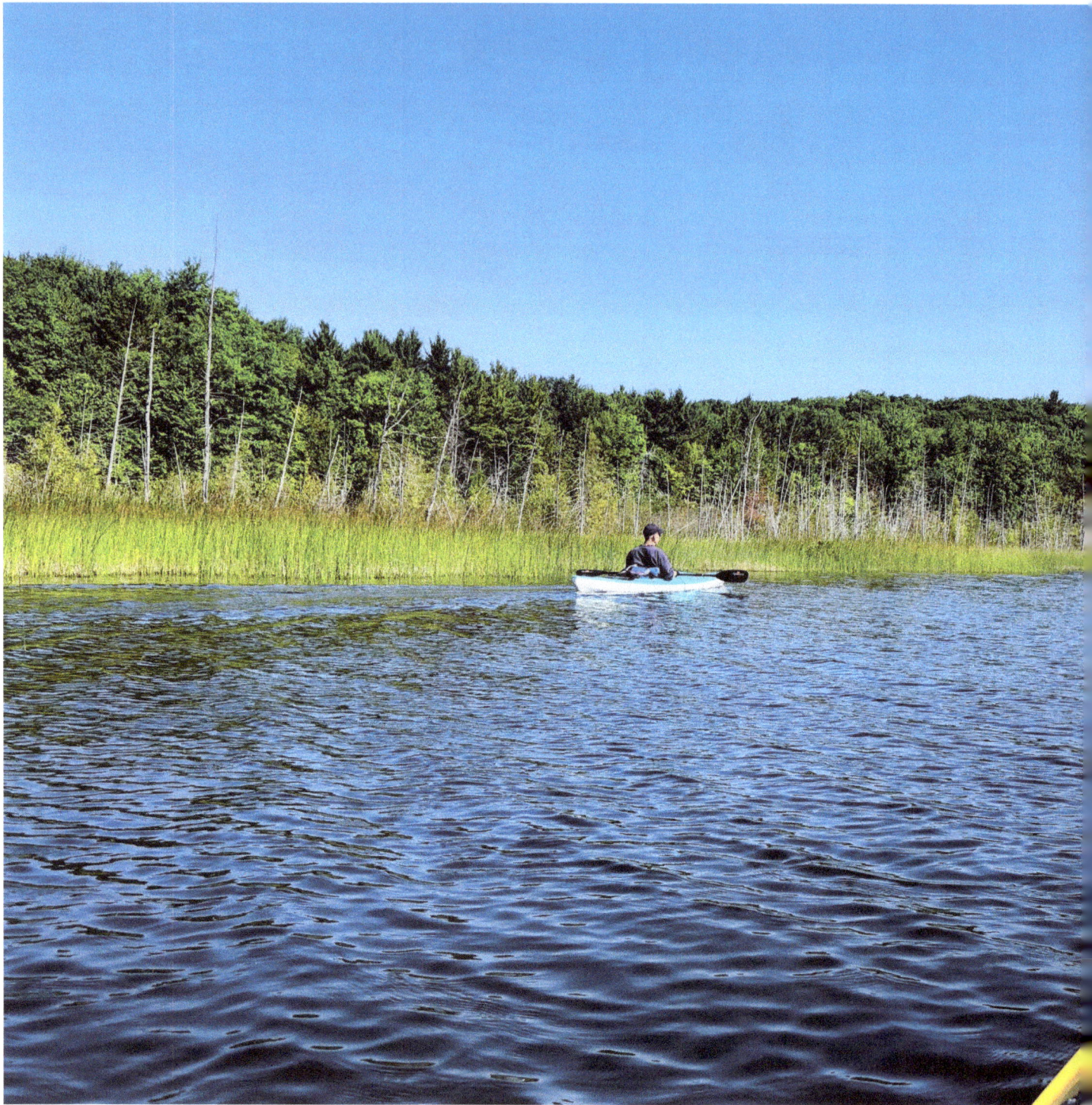

WOOLSEY LAKE

Also known as Mud Lake on many maps.

LOCATION: Woolsey Lake is located about 4 miles northeast of Northport and about 2 miles southwest of Lighthouse Point and about 1.5 miles directly east of Kehl Lake.

Directions to Woolsey Lake:

> » Take M-201 north out of Northport for 4 miles to Densmore Road. Turn left (north) on Densmore and go a short distance (300 feet) to the access road. Turn right on the access road (northeast) and travel 200 feet. There you will find a road loop area to park a vehicle and access the channel. I hope you have more luck in accessing Woolsey Lake than we did in 2018!

ACCESS: Although we weren't able to access Woolsey Lake on our first attempt in 2018, Larry and I were finally successful in doing so on July 31, 2019. Your best bet is the Densmore Road site. This is a carry in access down a 80-foot path through some light brush to reach a channel that leads to the lake. Because the water table was much higher, we were able to fairly easily launch our kayaks and paddle through a fairly narrow and shallow channel to the main lake. The effort proved to be well worth it as Woolsey Lake is truly a hidden gem with an undeveloped and unspoiled shoreline and an abundance of waterfowl and other birds to see. We saw several deer getting a morning drink of water as we paddled by. Our paddle around the lake on a calm and gorgeous day took us only an hour and ten minutes.

INFORMATION:

> » This is a larger lake than Kehl Lake, coming in at 145 acres and a shore-line of 2.5 miles.
>
> » Maps indicate that it is quite shallow with a marshy shoreline and a few tiny "islands".
>
> » It has no inlets but there is an outlet on the southern tip that extends one half mile southeast and into Lake Michigan

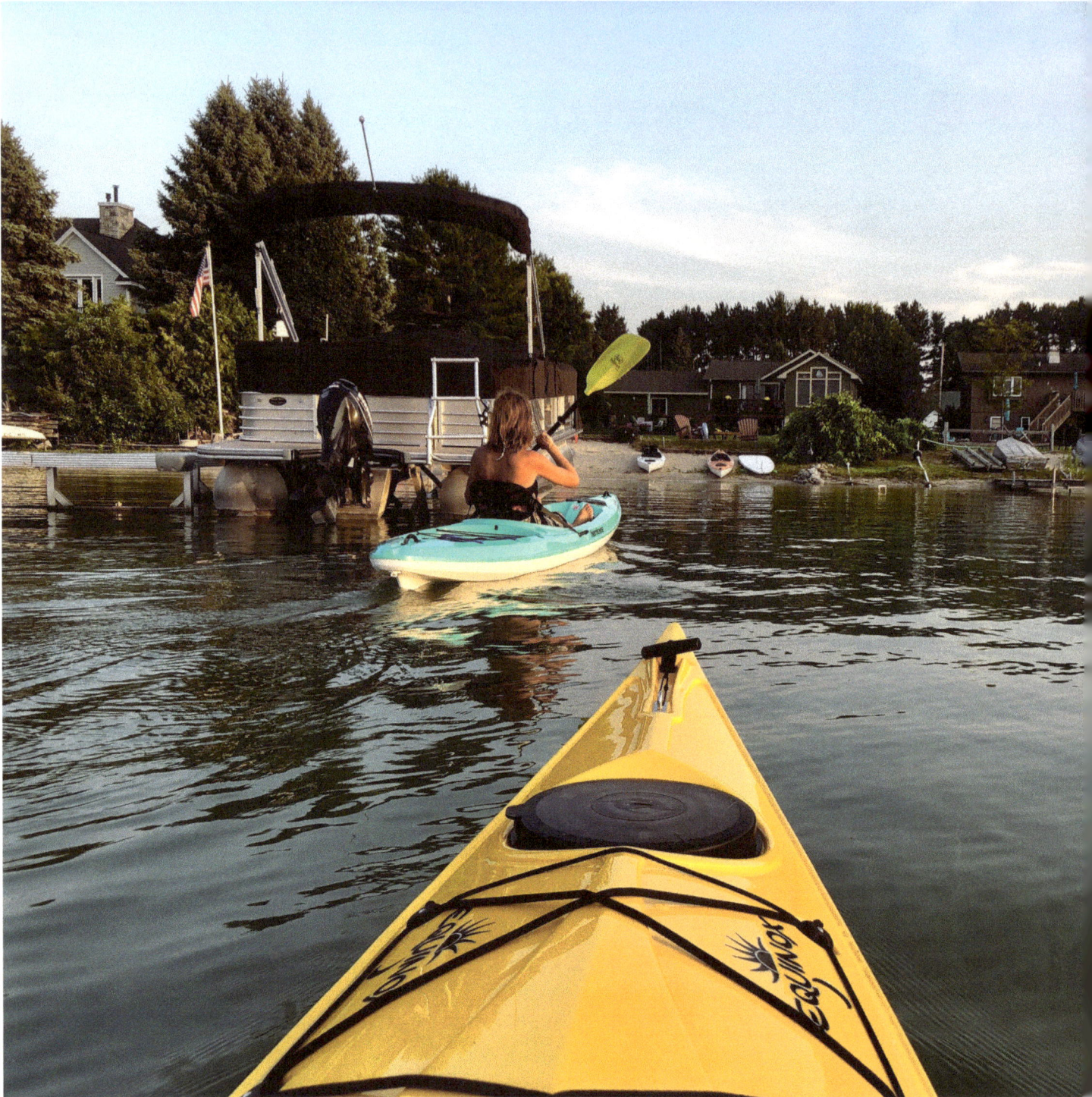

CEDAR LAKE

I've saved my favorite smaller lake in Leelanau until now. Cedar Lake is as unique as it is a beautiful, and is the closest to the urban area of Traverse City. Only two miles from the biggest city in northern Michigan, it can still feel like you are paddling in the Upper Peninsula or Canada — it is that unspoiled. How unusual to find a lake with a shoreline that is almost exactly like it was 100 years ago, and so close to Traverse City! And the colors of its water can be that brilliant turquoise, bluish-green, much like Torch Lake, Glen Lake or Key West — all just minutes from Traverse City!

LOCATION: Cedar Lake is in the extreme southeast corner of Leelanau County, just 2 miles north and west of Traverse City.

ACCESS: Cedar Lake has a boat launch at its south end. It is easily accessed off of Cherry Bend Road (County Road 633), just 0.3 miles from the stop light intersection of M-22. This site has a concrete ramp, parking, a dock and bathroom facilities.

INFORMATION:

» This is a small- to medium-sized lake of 252 acres with a shoreline of 3.9 miles.

» Cedar Lake has a maximum depth of 46 feet, located in the southeastern end, just north of the outlet to West Bay. The lake averages 35 feet deep in the south and about 25 feet deep in the north. All around the whole lake, there is a drop-off very near the shore.

» The main inlet is in the middle of the lake, on the western shore, and is labeled on maps as Cedar Creek — but it's called Hines Creek by longtime locals.

» Smaller inlets include two in the northwest corner and one in the southwest corner.

» There is an outflow channel called Cedar Creek that flows under M-22 and into West Grand Traverse Bay. Gladys Hill grew up on Cedar Lake and lived into her 90s. She shared stories of the history of Cedar Lake with me before she passed away, and said she remembered her mother talking about teams of horses working the creek, pulling scrapers to deepen the channel. The silting of Cedar Creek is a current issue for the lake and its residents.

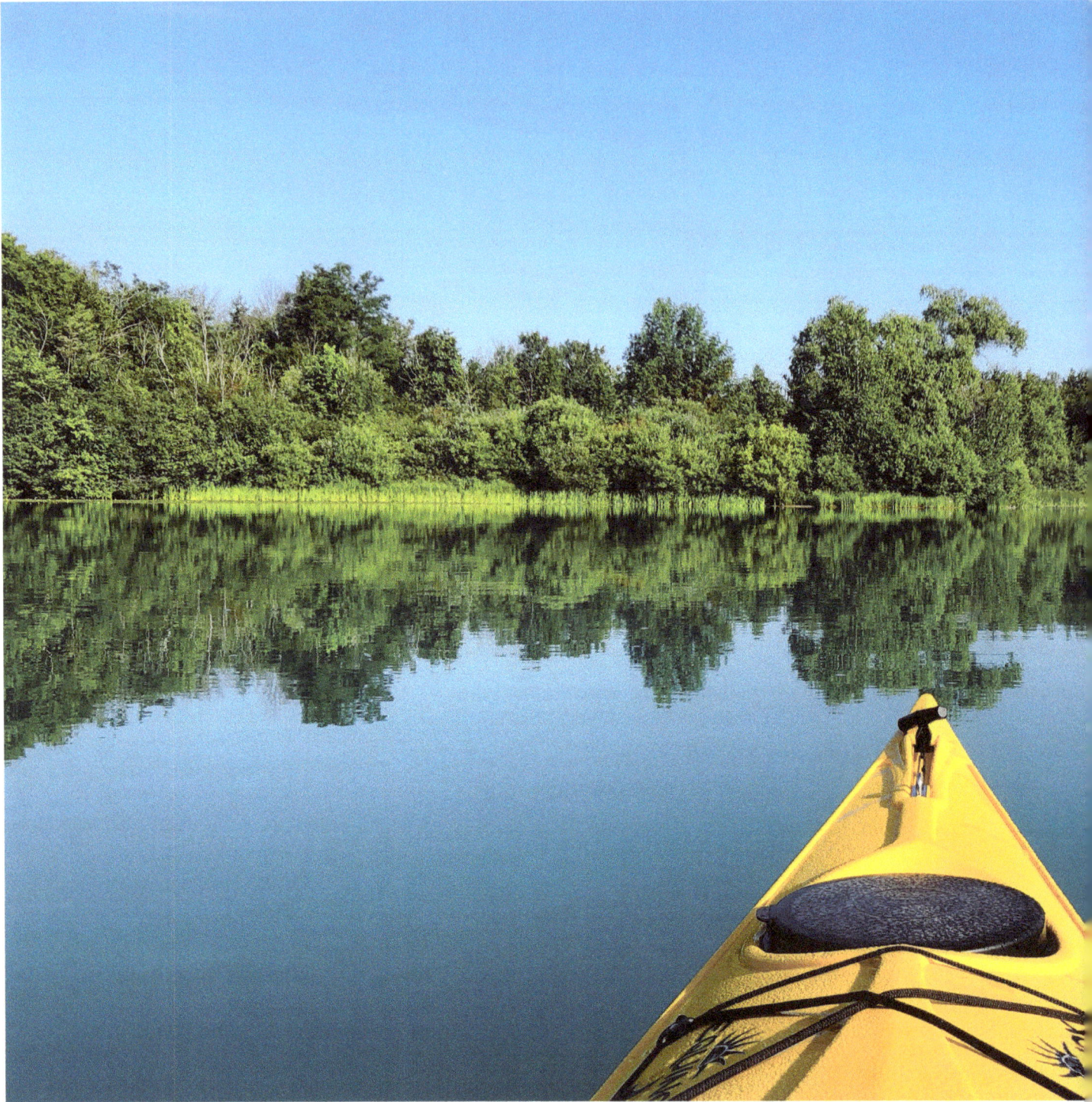

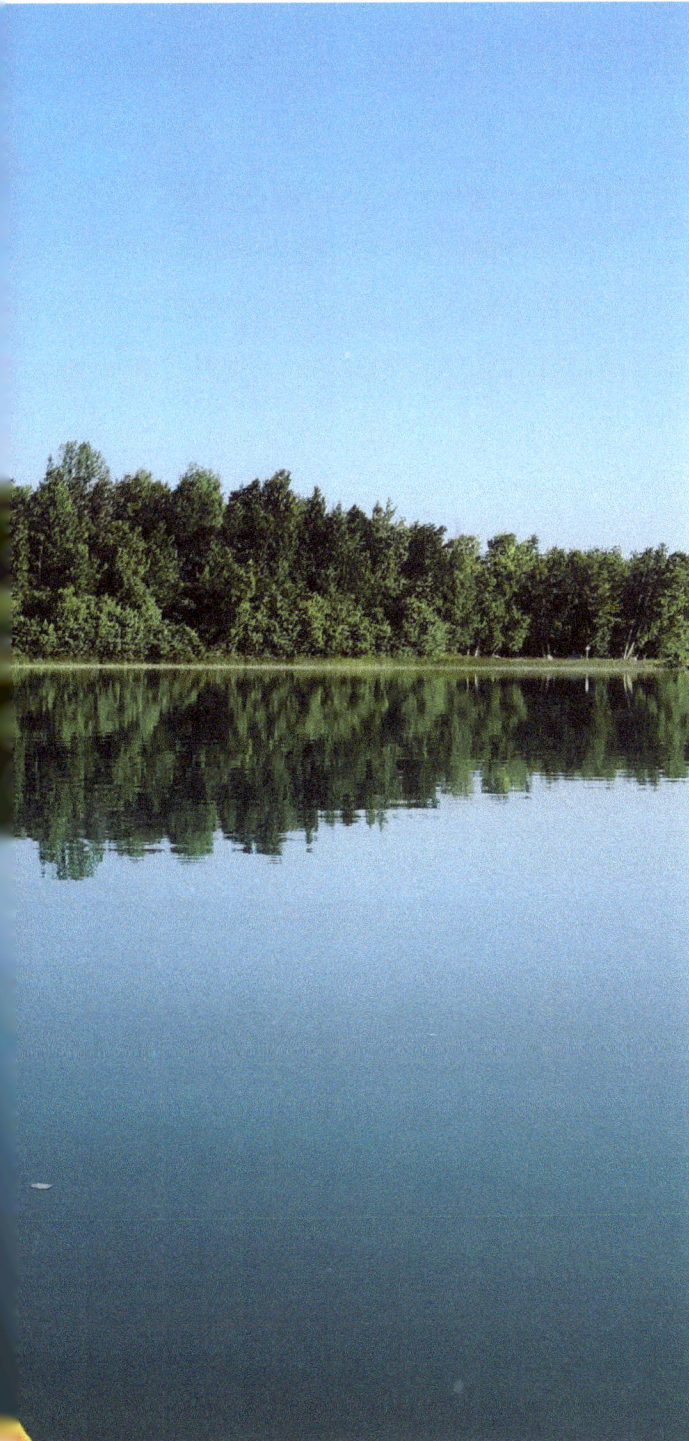

» In the early days, a canoe was available for those who needed to cross the stream on the trail from Leland to Suttons Bay. If the canoe was missing or was on the wrong side of the narrows, a strapping fellow named Napoleon Paulus would often offer to carry travelers on his shoulders, as he waded across the stream. At that time the Leland dam wasn't as high and the stream was fordable. Starting in 1864 a wooden bridge was built, the first of a series of bridges were built, replacing the need for Napoleon's job. An iron bridge with wood plank flooring was built around 1894 and that was replaced by a concrete bridge to its immediate north in the 1930s.

» From 1884 to 1921, a saw mill located on the east side of the narrows served as a fueling stop for the Tiger and the Leelanau, the two steamers who burned slab wood as they steamed their way back and forth from Leland to Fouch at the south end of South Lake Leelanau.

» If you would permit me a personal note— I would like to comment about the Babel family cottage on Lake Leelanau. My wife Mary's family has had a cottage on South Lake Leelanau's western shore since 1969. Built by Mary's dad, Larry Babel, the cottage is located midway between Kelenskes Point and the Leelanau Pines Resort. The cottage has been a great spot for many family memories— and a great place to take a kayak paddle and explore the southern sections of this awesome lake. Be sure to call ahead for reservations to use our launch site.

» By 1863 there were two tugs and several scows taking logs and cordwood from lumbering operations around the lake to Leland.

» Cedar Lake was the source ice for Traverse City in the days prior to refrigeration. There are many pilings, especially on the southern end of the lake, which were once the wooden ramps used to slide the cut ice out of the frozen lake. The ice was then stored under sawdust in shanties before being shipped to customers in Traverse City.

» Most of the yellow bricks that built the downtown Traverse City buildings and most of the State Hospital (now the Grand Traverse Commons) came from the hills between Cedar Lake and Grand Traverse Bay. From the water, you can see where the Markham Brickworks got the clay and marl. A small gauge train was used to transport the bricks from Greilickville to Traverse City.

» The Traverse City to Suttons Bay TART Trail runs along the western side of Cedar Lake. This bike path uses the old railroad tracks that connected Traverse City and Northport.

» There is a floating fishing/observation dock on the northwest corner of Cedar Lake. This dock is part of the DeYoung Natural Area, a 145-acre park that includes a farm and homestead dating back to 1870, and a mile of shoreline on Cedar Lake — the greatest amount of protected shoreline of any inland lake in Leelanau county. The DeYoung Natural Area was named for Louis DeYoung, who helped develop the cherry industry in the area and died at the age of 104. His dream was to protect and preserve his farm and property.

» The Pathfinder School dock, near the middle of the eastern shore, is a landmark for kayakers. It is used in the summer for the school's swimming instruction program.

» The Cedar Lake Ski Course is located in a protected bay in the middle and western part of the lake. For years, there was a wooden ski jump (rumored to have been used in a Tim Allen "Home Improvement" episode) in this spot. Currently, it is the location of a slalom ski course used by water ski enthusiasts nearly every morning and evening. Kayakers need to be aware that they're sharing the lake with these ski boats and skiers.

» Cedar Lake is a popular fishing lake. In the spring, you can see small-mouth bass and suckers laying eggs — and guarding the eggs. One of the rarest fish I've ever seen from my kayak was spotted on Cedar Lake: a hybrid between a muskie and a pike, known as a "Tiger Muskie." According to my deceased neighbor Gladys, the Tiger Muskies were planted in the 1940s and 1950s. Supposedly they can't reproduce naturally, but I've seen a few of these huge fish in the shallows in the evening. One of Gladys' stories was of an elderly neighbor who wanted to catch one of these monsters before he died. She reported that he did finally catch one, but unfortunately, his wish fulfillment caused a heart attack and he died shortly after landing his dream fish. I guess that there are worse ways to die.

» There is a short creek that flows out of the southeast end of Cedar Lake to West Grand Traverse Bay that can be paddled to the dam that is located just east of the bridge on M-22. This little creek runs behind the Leelanau Art Center.

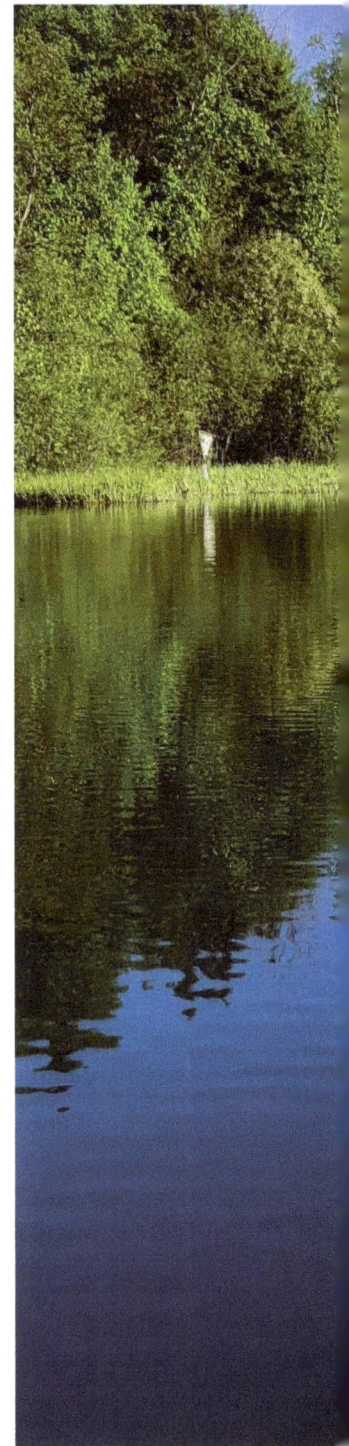

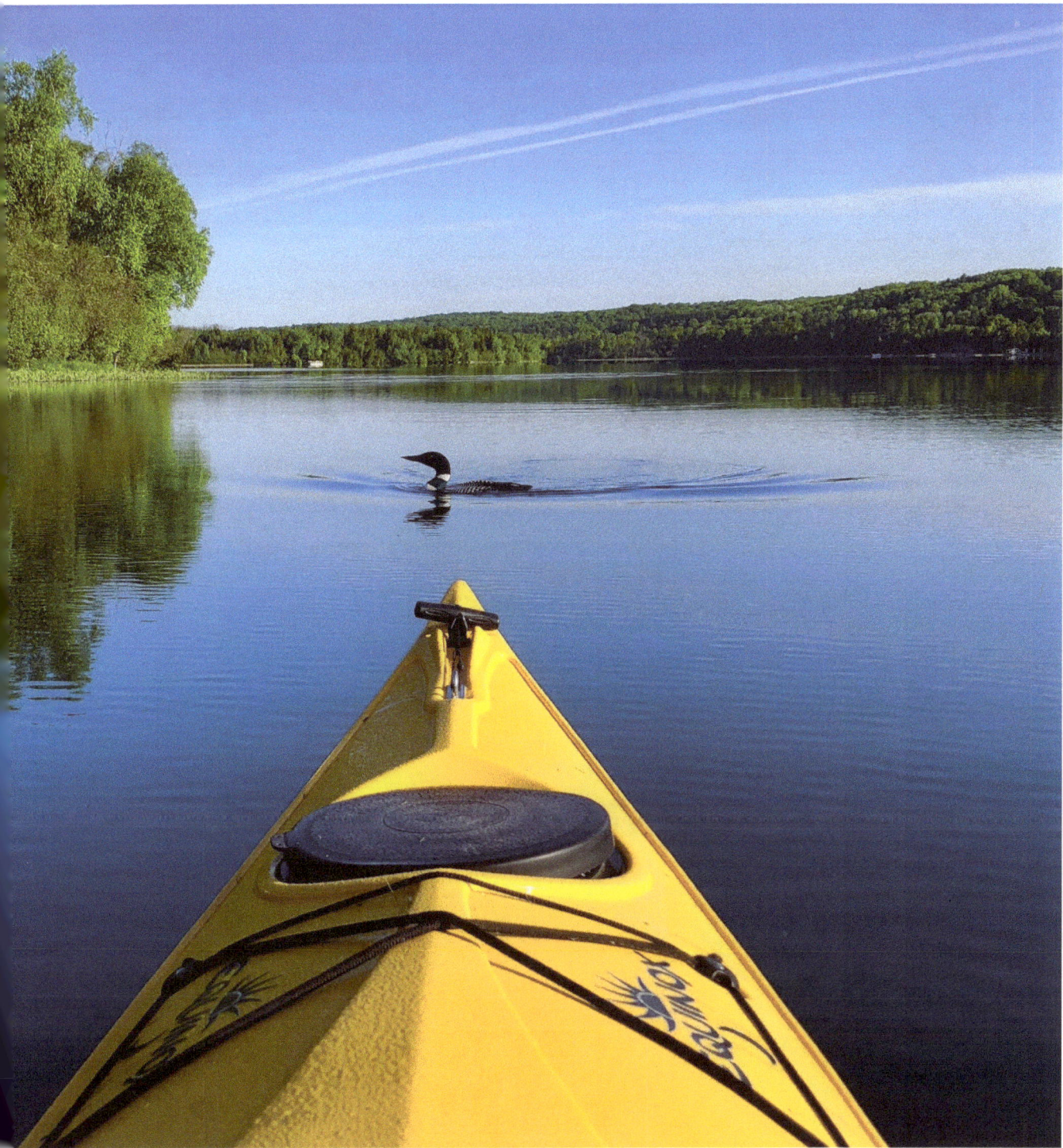

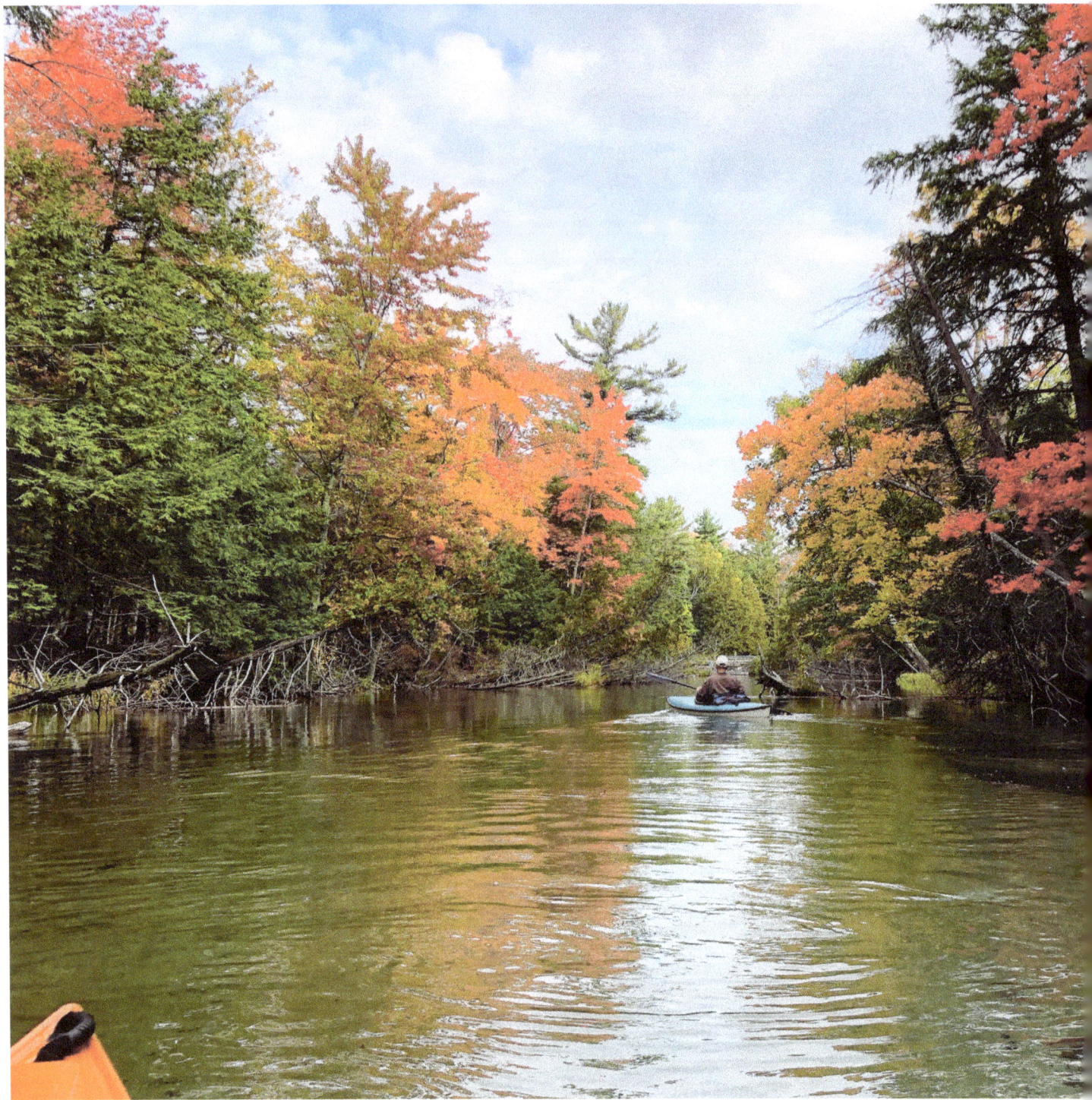

PADDLING LEELANAU'S RIVERS

The Leelanau Peninsula has three rivers that are suitable for kayaking — the Leland River, the Cedar River and the Crystal River. We've done less kayaking on the rivers than the lakes, but some paddlers specialize on rivers and I can see why — river kayaking can be great fun. It's also a great alternative when conditions are too windy for paddling on more open waters.

Here is where and how we kayaked the rivers in Leelanau, and what it looked like.

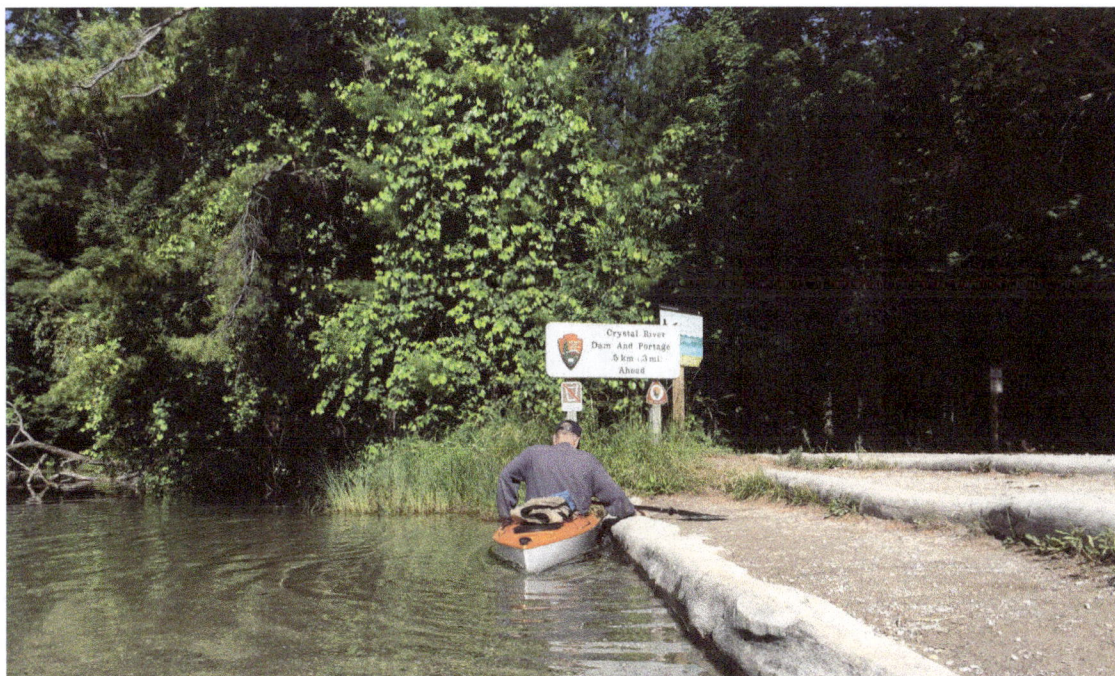

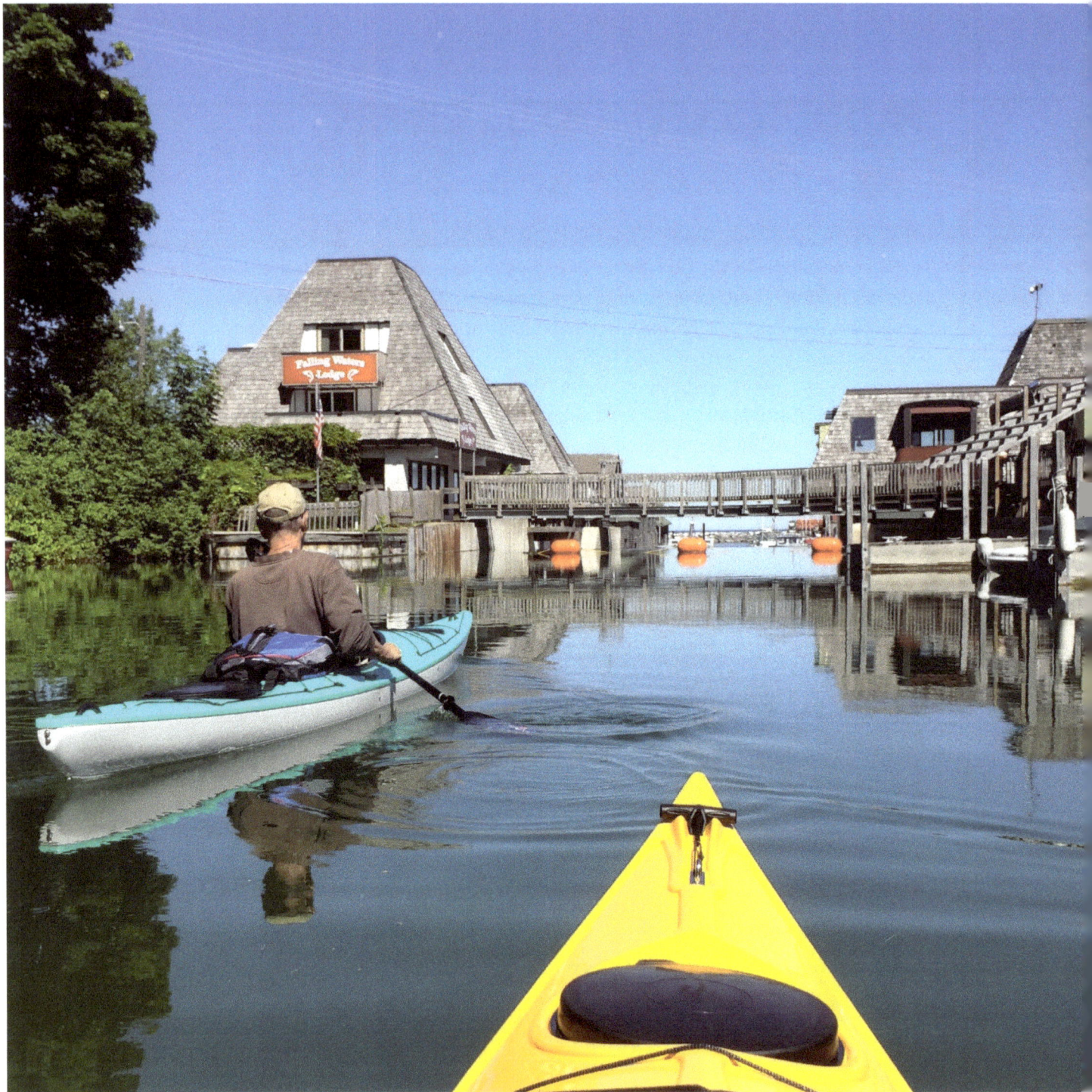

THE LELAND RIVER

The Leland River is also called The Carp River on some maps, and the Carp is what the locals call it. This river is the mildest and shortest of the three main rivers in Leelanau County. It's also only about a mile in length. And, it can be busy. You're likely to find yourself sharing the river with lots of motorized boats, plus pontoon boats and even some classic wooden boats. Once, we saw an amphibious car/boat "driving" down the river.

Besides the boat traffic, there are many other sites to see as you paddle this delightful and short river. There are houses big and small, old and new. On the east bank, check out the Stander Marine operation. There are several community buildings, like the Leelanau Historical Museum and the Leland Township Library. You could also land your kayak near the Bluebird Restaurant & Bar, have a meal, then explore the sights and sounds of Fishtown. I enjoy paddling right up to the dam that overlooks Fishtown and stopping for a moment to take in the views.

LOCATION: The Leland River runs right through the town of Leland.

ACCESS: We've used some of the nearby launches on North Lake Leelanau to get to this river, but the easiest and best access would be the DNR site on River Street, right next to the Bluebird Restaurant & Bar on River Street.

COMMENTS:

» Although this is an easy river for kayaking, it's advisable to keep an eye on where the deeper channel of the river runs to avoid hitting the bottom.

» It took us only about 25 minutes to leisurely paddle from the Chandler Street dead end launch on North Lake Leelanau to the Cedar River to the dam above Fishtown.

» One of the biggest structures is the Riverview Inn built in the Victorian style.

» Opposite the DNR docks, you will see much more modern buildings. One of them is the Leland Public Library and another is the Leelanau Historical Museum.

» Keep an eye out for a classic wooden boat going by. Many wooden boats are docked in the protected slips at Stander Marine on the east side of the river.

» Larry and I have paddled this section three times, and we definitely will be back.

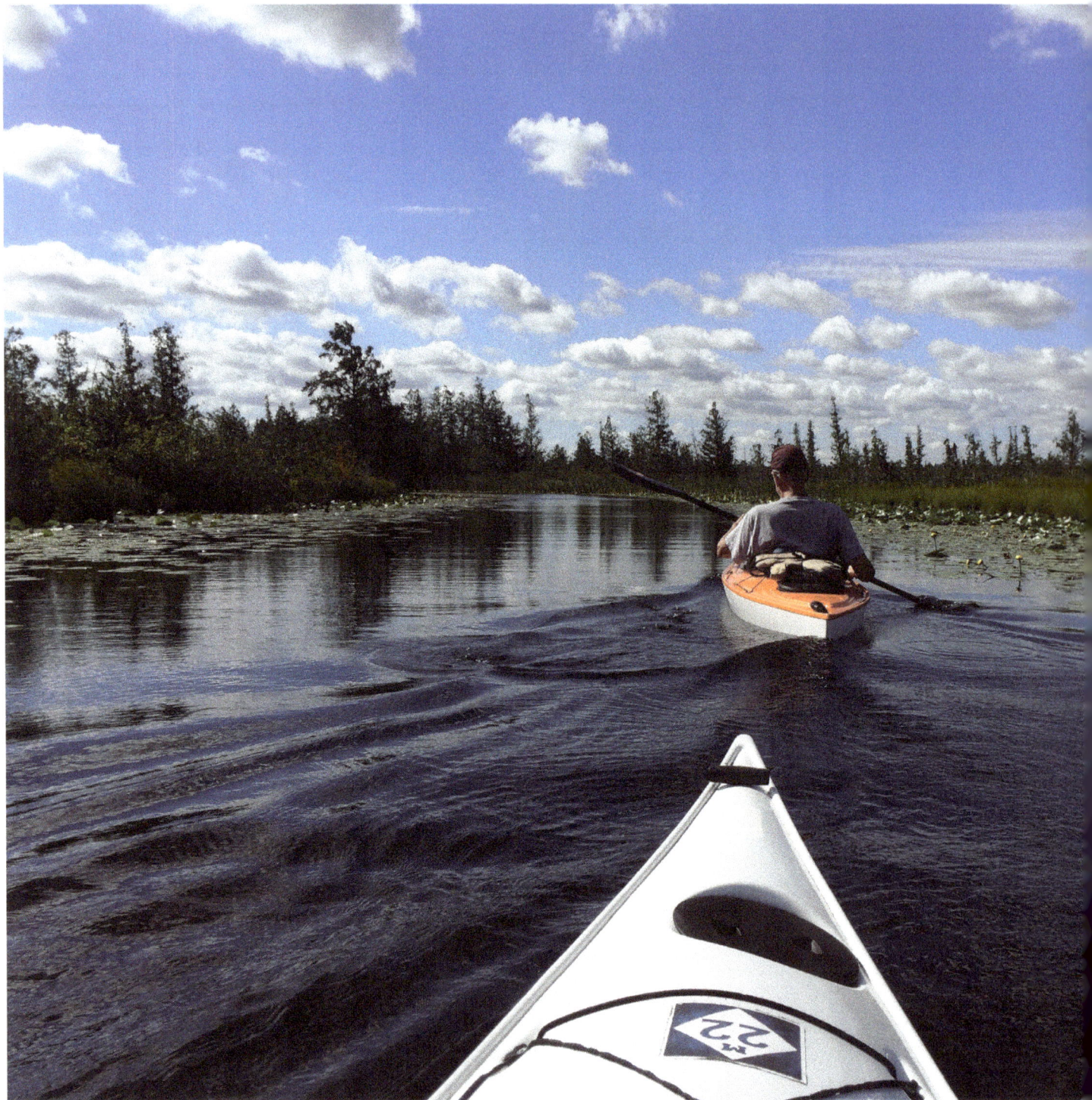

THE CEDAR RIVER

The Cedar is a slow river that meanders through the edge of the village of Cedar and on into a very large wetlands known locally as Solon Swamp. From the swamp, the river winds its way into the heart of Leelanau County, finally entering South Lake Leelanau at its southwest corner. The distance from a launch at the village of Cedar to the opening to South Lake Leelanau is about 4 miles. Along the way, you will see a variety of birds, animals and vegetation. We saw dozens of muskrats and a few beavers. We also saw many species of birds, including song sparrows, kingbirds, marsh wrens, kingfishers and green herons.

A paddle on this river most likely means making a round trip, as there is no close landing or solid shore where the river enters South Lake Leelanau. This means that there will be some paddling against the gentle flow of the river. Also, it was windy one of the days we paddled, and that increased the difficulty just a bit. We had parked our vehicle at Perins Landing, and had some trouble negotiating the open southern end of Lake Leelanau. Paddle time that day was about 1.5 hours from Cedar to Perins Landing.

Like so many Leelanau spots, the Cedar River has a local name, Victoria Creek.

LOCATION: The Cedar River is located just north of the village of Cedar.

ACCESS: We used the Cedar Village Park to get on the river. This park is located just north of the main intersection in Cedar. There is a small ramp, ample parking, picnic facilities and restrooms available.

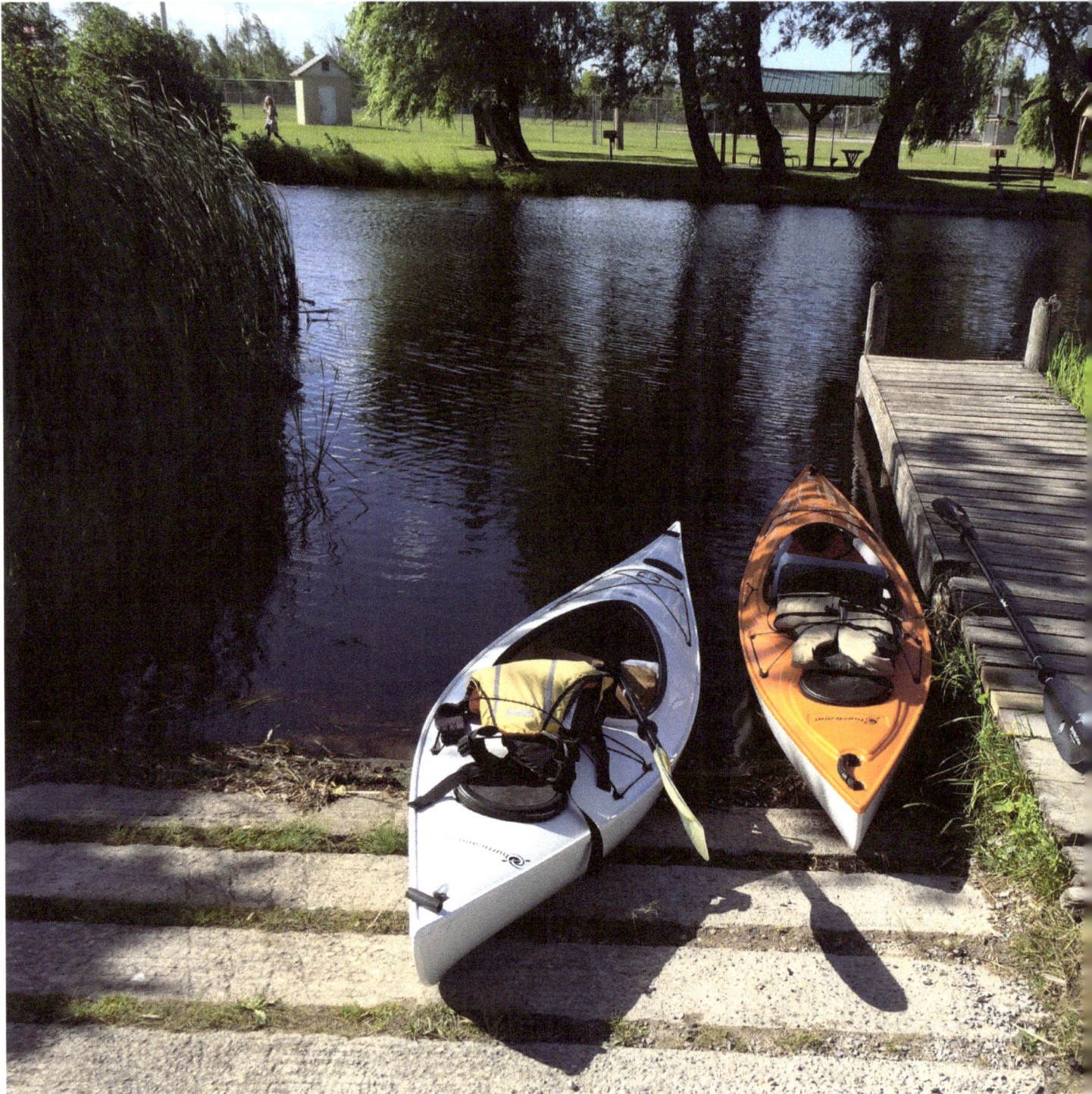

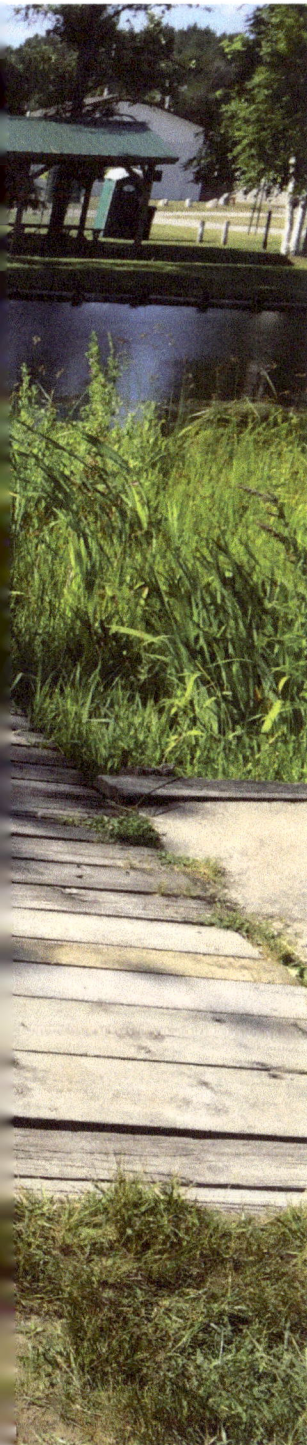

COMMENTS:

» Larry and I have done both round trips and one-way trips on the Cedar River. For a one-way trip, you can drop a second vehicle at either Perin's Landing at the south end of Lake Leelanau or at Solon Township Park about a mile north of the river's mouth. Solon Township Park is on County Road 643 (Lake Shore Drive).

» My science teacher friends tell me that the Cedar River flows through a "fen," not a swamp. Fens are different than swamps or bogs in that they are less acidic, have higher nutrient levels and can support a more diversified plant and animal community. This fen has many grasses, lily pads, mosses and sedges. And yes, Fenway Park is named for a fen in Boston.

» The wetlands here are part of the Cedar River Preserve (The Leelanau Land Conservancy). It is only accessible by boat or kayak. According to the Conservancy website, this area is actually several ecosystems and many micro-habitats — including fen, shrub scrub and aquatic systems. There is an index based on Michigan Natural Features that ranks an area's importance by the number of significant native plants and flowers. It's called the FQI (floristic quality index), and any number greater than 35 is significant, and indicates a significant native biodiversity. The FQI for the Cedar Preserve is 91.1. There are 262 native plant species in the Cedar River Preserve's 480 acres! The wetland complex is also very important to the health of Lake Leelanau. It's interesting that there has been little or no human impact on this area, other than some cedars that were lumbered over 100 years ago. Not many areas in Michigan can say that.

» We observed many muskrats, mink and lots of beautiful yellow pond lilies on our paddles on the Cedar River. Sandhill cranes also are common just north of the wetlands.

» We haven't tried it, but you can paddle the opposite direction from the access site in Cedar, going upstream. It is possible to paddle about a half mile against the gentle flow of Victoria Creek (Cedar River).

» The village of Cedar was founded in 1885 by the lumberman Benjamin Boughey. The Manistee and North-Eastern Railroad railroad came through in 1892. Its first name was Cedar City, given by the Sullivan Lumber Company which had a small cedar shingle mill there.

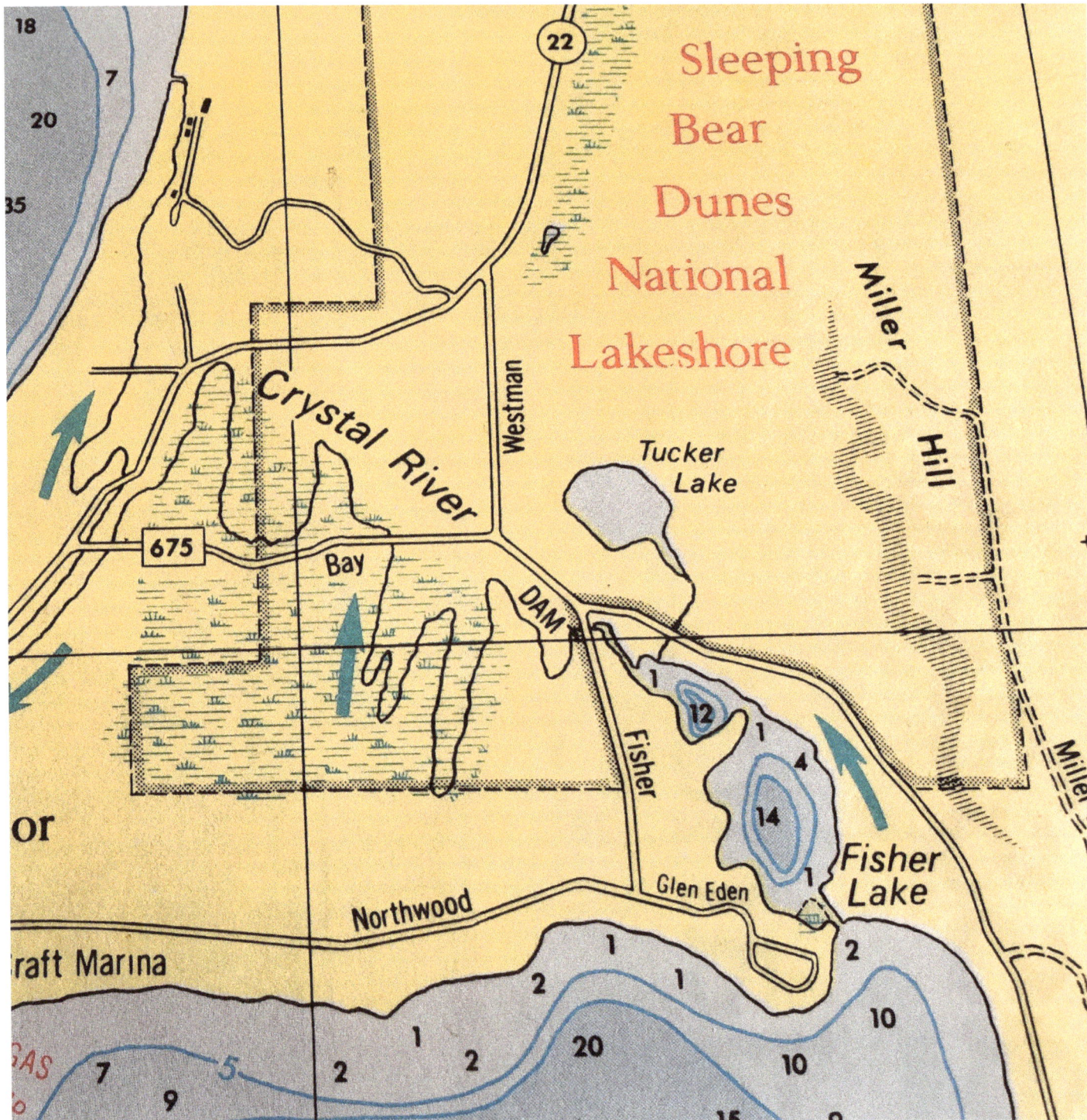

18

7

20

35

22

Sleeping
Bear
Dunes
National
Lakeshore

Miller Hill

Crystal River

Westman

Tucker
Lake

675

Bay

DAM

Fisher

Miller

1

12

1

4

14

1

Fisher
Lake

or

Glen Eden

2

Northwood

1

1

2

raft Marina

1

1

2

10

GAS

7

5

2

1

2

20

10

15

9

10

2

THE CRYSTAL RIVER

The Crystal River is one of our favorite paddling destinations. You start in a very wild, almost eerie stretch of the river with huge trees — some hanging precariously over the river — then move to a more open, yet still undeveloped stretch that becomes a more developed area before ending in Glen Arbor itself. It might as well be called "The Crooked River," as it flows 6.4 miles back and forth, to cover only 1.4 miles as the crow flies. This river is a great alternative paddle when the winds are blowing, as it is well protected.

The Glen Arbor area was hard hit by the wind storm of 2015, but crews worked hard to keep the river cleared. Even so, be alert to fallen and / or partially cleared trees.

Larry and I have kayaked this beautiful river four times, and highly recommend that you do so, too. However, it's also our recommendation that you paddle The Crystal during non-peak times (not July or August) — unless you like crowds. Much of Crystal River flows through the National Lakeshore, so depending on where you park, you may need a park pass.

LOCATION: The Crystal River is located just north of Big Glen Lake and Fisher Lake and just south of Sleeping Bear Bay and Glen Arbor.

ACCESS: We used the National Lakeshore's Fisher Road access. This site is just north of Fisher Lake, near the intersection of Dunn's Farm Road (County Road 675) and Fisher Road. A park pass is required to park a vehicle here. It took us about 2 hours to paddle the 5 miles from put-in to take out.

- The other option is to use the small, sandy landing near Bay Street in Glen Arbor, close to the mouth of the river. Bay Street becomes Dunn's Farm Road (County Road 675) as it crosses the bridge. Limited parking is available on Bay Street.

COMMENTS:

» The Crystal can be quite shallow, even with a dam regulating its depth, and we've paddled when we had to pay close attention to the main channel of the river. I also decided to use one of my older kayaks on this river, as there are plenty of stones and fallen trees to negotiate over and around.

» There are several required portages because of road bridges. The last one, on West County Road 675, can be particularly tricky to re-enter the water. "Shooting the tube" under one of the bridges is pretty cool, but one time the river was so low that we opted to portage that spot. Of the three tubes, the one on the left is usually the best.

» In the fall, the Crystal can be full of runs of salmon and trout — and the numbers can be amazing. Several of the salmon we observed must have been close to 20 pounds, and a few of them actually "torpedoed" my kayak. I managed to survive.

» We have also seen many bald eagles in flight or perched in trees, looking for their next meal. Their screech is something to hear!

» On our last paddle on The Crystal, we were about halfway around when we heard a screech behind us and a great blue heron flew right past and landed just ahead of us on the river. I think we were bothering his search for breakfast. He stood his ground as we paddled by him.

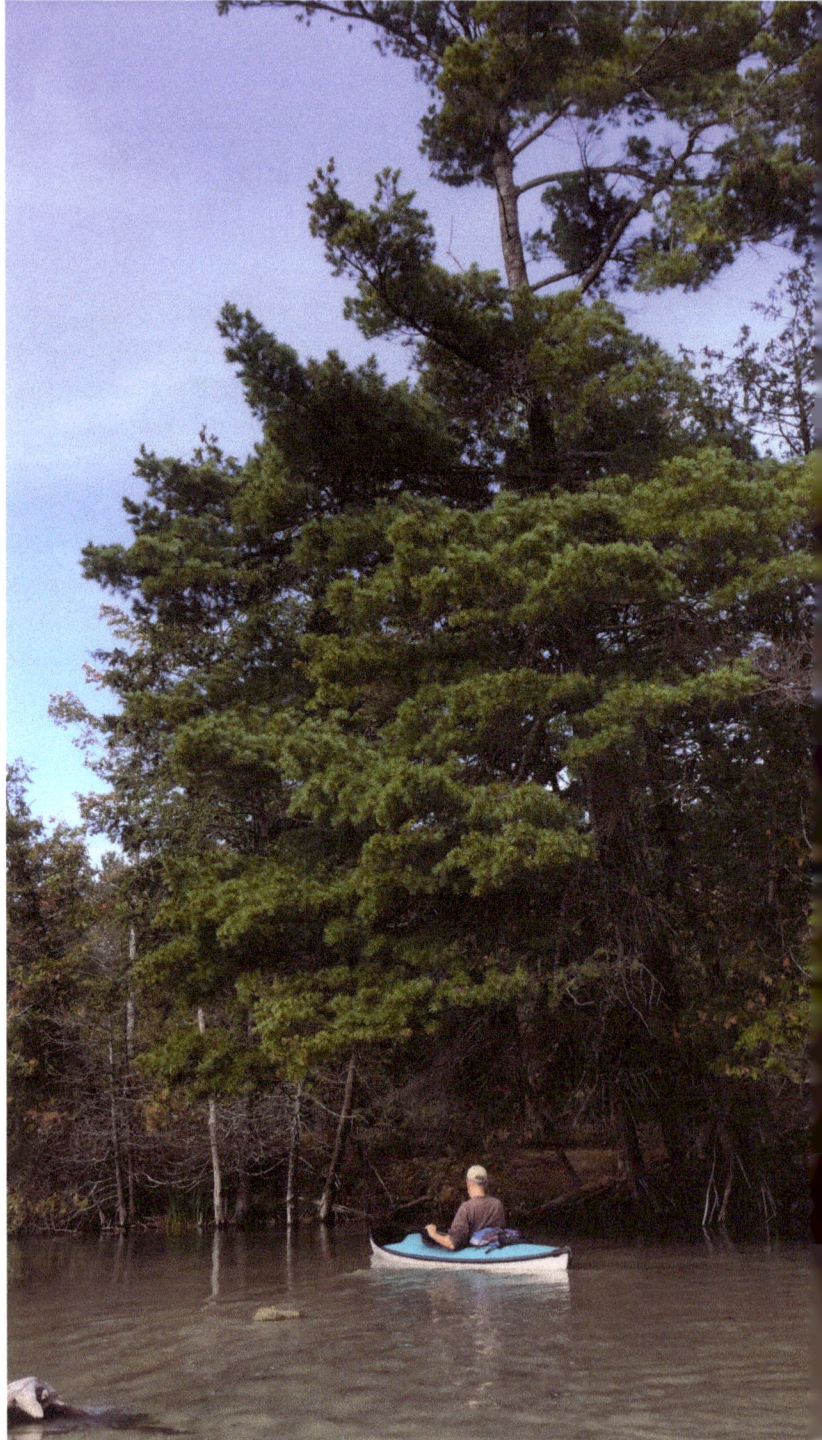

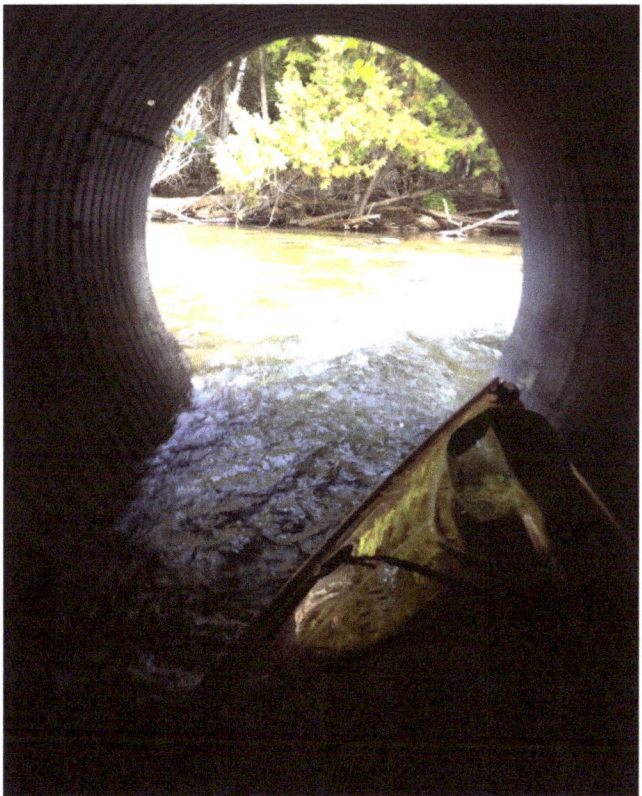
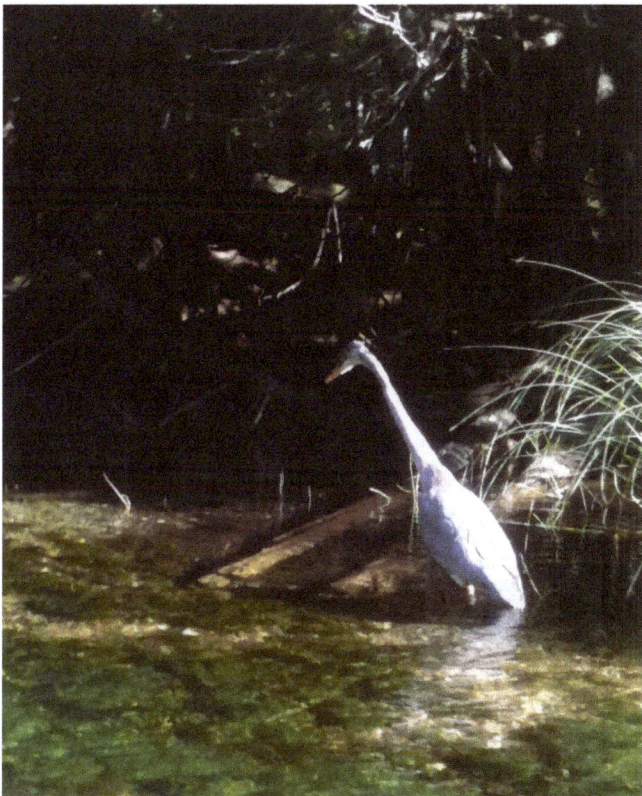
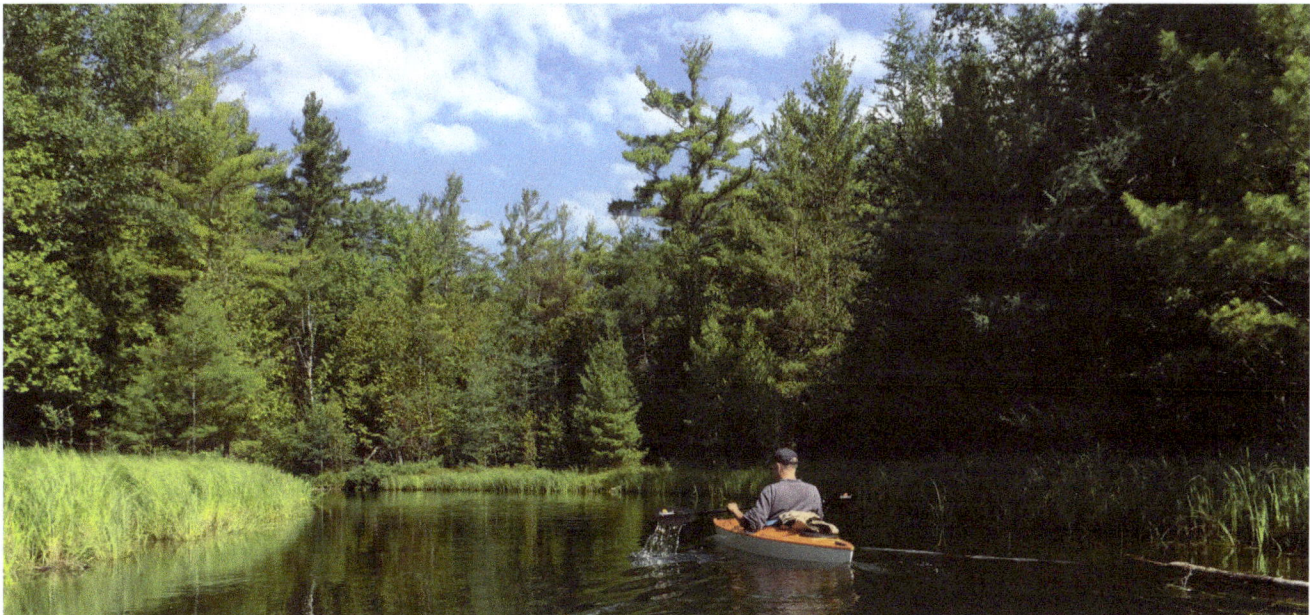

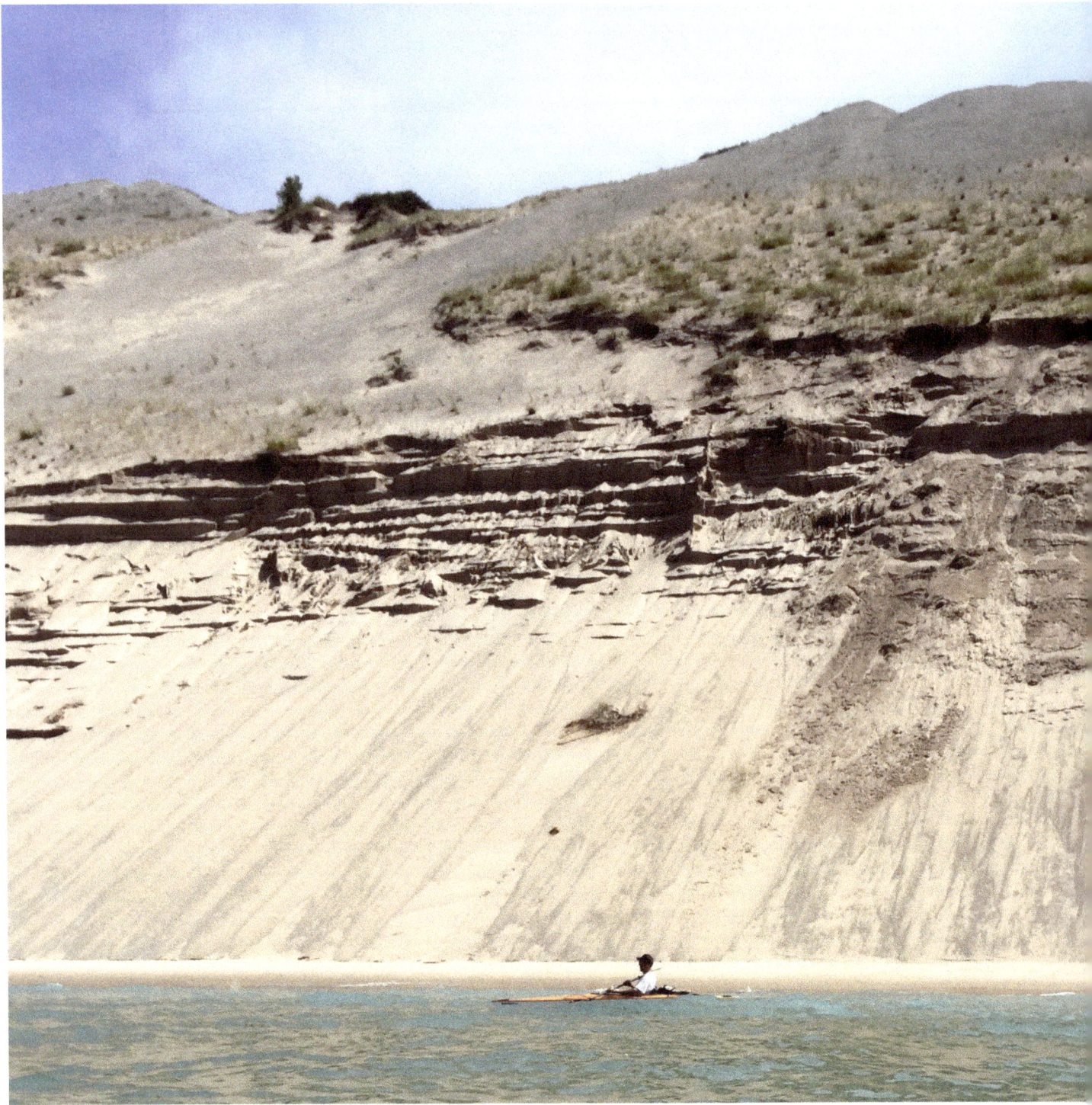

PRACTICAL MATTERS

THIS IS A LIST OF SOME OF OUR EQUIPMENT:

- » Kayaks: Hurricane Santee 12.6; Hurricane Santee 13.6; Hurricane Sojourn 13.5; Eddyline Equinox 14 ft.
- » Paddles: Werner Skagit; Werner Camano; Aqua-bound Manta Ray
- » Kayak spray skirt: Eddyline
- » Life Jacket: Patagonia Kayaking Jacket
- » Camera: iPhone 6 and iPhone 8
- » Sleeping Bear Dunes National Lakeshore Park Pass
- » Michigan State Park Pass (Leelanau Lighthouse State Park)
- » Kayak Racks: Yakima

SAFETY TIPS:

» **Avoid dangerous conditions on the water.** I always check several sources for the weather, and we pick our days very carefully — especially when we are planning on going out on Lake Michigan. Wind direction and wind speeds are crucially important. My sources for weather conditions include the Weather Channel App on my iPad, the Weather Page in the Traverse City *Record-Eagle* and the local weather on TV stations 9&10 and 7&4. Obviously, the lower the wind the better, and going with the wind is better than going into it. Also, since we're paddling a peninsula, it can be an advantage to paddle the side opposite from where the wind is blowing. Be extremely conservative on the Big Lake. If you are in doubt, choose a more protected river, lake or bay, and come back on a better day. Keep an eye on the sky. Conditions can change and forecasts can be less than accurate.

» **Bring the right equipment and supplies.** A longer kayak is better on Lake Michigan. We used kayaks in the 12–14-foot lengths. Sit-on-top kayaks are popular, and would be fine on smaller lakes. Our preference is kayaks that have sit-inside cockpits. This type of kayak gives more protection from waves and wind and even the sun. Other equipment choices include sunglasses, sunscreen, bottles of water, something to bail out your kayak (a sponge or bilge pump), a baggie or waterproof container for a cell phone. Wear a life jacket or a PFD. I know many of the pictures show us not wearing them in calm, warm water situations, but we have recently decided to wear them at all times on Lake Michigan and everywhere early or late in the season, or when the water is colder or when the winds pick up. I am in favor of the proposed idea that all kayakers must wear life jackets at all times when on the Great Lakes.

- » **Don't paddle alone.** Some of the places we paddled are very remote and two people make for a safer trip — and good conversations!

- » **Don't drink alcohol and paddle.** Water is all you need to drink.

- » **It is safer to stay close to shore**, and you can see so much more. A kayak brought to shore is much more easy to bail and to re-enter.

- » **Know your skill level** and choose a trip and conditions that match your experience. Pick locations that are most protected from the winds. Because of colder water temperatures and the risks of hypothermia, it is more dangerous earlier in the season and later in the fall, so be even more cautious at those times of the year.

HOW TO PREPARE:

- » Conditions are usually better for kayaking earlier in morning or later in the evening. Winds tend to be calmer, and there are less boats and jet skis at those times. Larry and I would usually leave for a day trip around 8:30 AM , and hit the water between 9:00 and 10:00 AM. Our time on the water would range from around 3 or 4 hours. Usually, this results in about a 7–10-mile paddle.

- » Eat and drink something (but not too much) before paddling. I usually have a cup of coffee and a banana. It is always good if there are bathrooms or Porta Potties where you launch — if you know what I mean.

- » When we first began paddling, we would use only one vehicle to transport our kayaks to our launch. That is fine — but however far you paddle, eventually you have to turn around and go back. Eventually, we evolved into taking two vehicles — driving one car to our end-of- trip destination, leaving it and heading to our launch location. This allows us to paddle twice as far and have the winds at our backs (if the winds stay as predicted).

- » Clothing choices are important. On hot and sunny days, I try to wear a broad-brimmed hat or baseball cap, sunglasses, light clothing, shorts, flip flops and plenty of sunscreen. I usually pack rain gear in one of my kayak compartments. Next year, I will be packing a whistle and a first aid kit. On cooler days (or cooler mornings), I bring or wear a sweatshirt. I also bring a towel to use as needed. (Towels can cover your legs from the direct rays of the sun and be a good place to rest your cell phone.)

- » One of the most important pieces of advice I can suggest is to buy as good a paddle as you can afford. Both Larry and I speak from experience — a good paddle makes a "good paddle" (especially at our age). Look for a paddle that is lightweight and top quality. Good paddles are pricey, but they are one of the most important things you can invest in for longer trips. Believe us, your shoulders and your arms will thank you the next day!

» If you get to a destination and the winds and waves are more than you expected, have a Plan B. More than once, we have arrived at a site on Lake Michigan, only to see the lake in a mood we would rather not experience first hand. Fortunately, it's easy to make the short trip to an inland lake or river in Leelanau county.

» Get a good set of maps. I use several maps, as well as the Google Maps app on my iPhone. I enjoy the old set of maps made by "Mapping Unlimited" because they have the depths of the bodies of water. I also use the free maps of Leelanau county made by "Michigan Maps" that are available around the area. These maps have more updated roads and launch sites, and the price is right.

» We try to stay in decent shape throughout the year. I try to remember that I'm working out while shoveling snow in my driveway during the winter!

» Have something to mark your take-out destination if it is not clearly identifiable from the water. Some of the access sites can be very difficult to locate from offshore. We use an orange and white winter driveway stick.

» Using your cellphone for taking pictures will drain the battery very quickly. I have found that turning off apps and shutting off the phone manually will extend the charge. Also, keeping it out of the direct sunlight is advised.

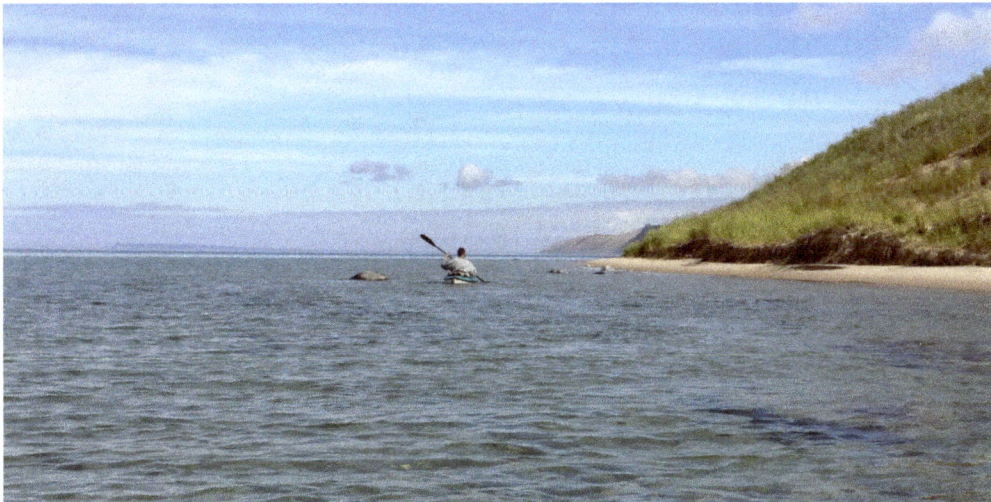

SOME OF THE BOOKS THAT WERE VERY HELPFUL IN THE WRITING OF THIS BOOK INCLUDE:

- *A Guide to the Rivers and Lakes of Grand Traverse and Leelanau Counties, Michigan*, By Jim Stamm, 2015.

- *Destination: Leelanau, Boats Sailing Leelanau Waters 1835-1900*, by Claudia D. Goudschaal, The Old Scott Farm, 2009.

- *Wood Boats of Leelanau: A Photographic Journal*, by John C. Mitchell, The Leelanau Historical Society, 2007.

- *Geology*, compiled by Kerry Kelly, A Publication of Friends of Sleeping Bear Dunes, 2011.

- *Ghost Towns*, compiled by Kerry Kelly, A Publication of the Friends of Sleeping Bear Dunes, 2014.

- *The Last Ice Age and the Leelanau Peninsula*, by Thomas H. Hooker, Dog Ear Publishing, 2014.

LEELANAU HISTORY AND MUSEUMS

- Empire Area Museum; 11544 LaCore Road, Empire, Mi 49630
  (231) 326-5568 • empiremimuseum.org

- Leelanau Historical Society; 203 E. Cedar Street, Leland, MI 49654
  (231) 256-7475 • leelanauhistory.org

- Omena Historical Society and Museum; 5045 N. West Bay Shore Drive, Omena Mi 49674
  (231) 326-4726 • nps.gov

THE MAPS THAT WERE VERY HELPFUL IN OUR PLANNING FOR OUR KAYAK TRIPS AND IN DEVELOPING THIS BOOK INCLUDE:

- The Leelanau County map located opposite the Contents page was used by permission of Michigan Maps, Inc., (Mark Stone), P.O. Box 885 Elk Rapids, Michigan, 49629.

- The other maps were used with permission of of *Mapping Unlimited*, (Butch and Linda Hoogerhyde), 6235 Crystal Springs Road, Bellaire, Michigan, 49615.

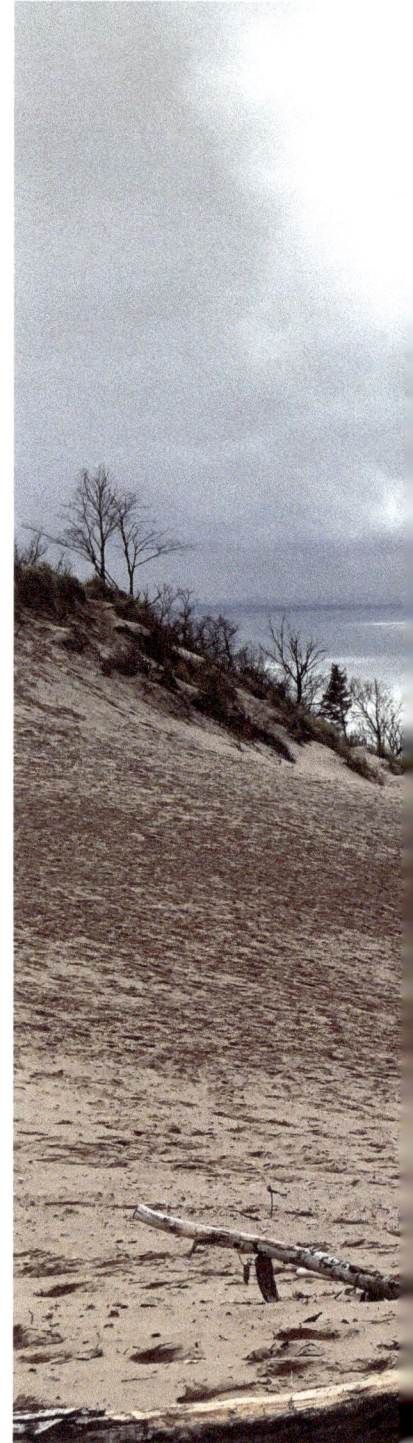

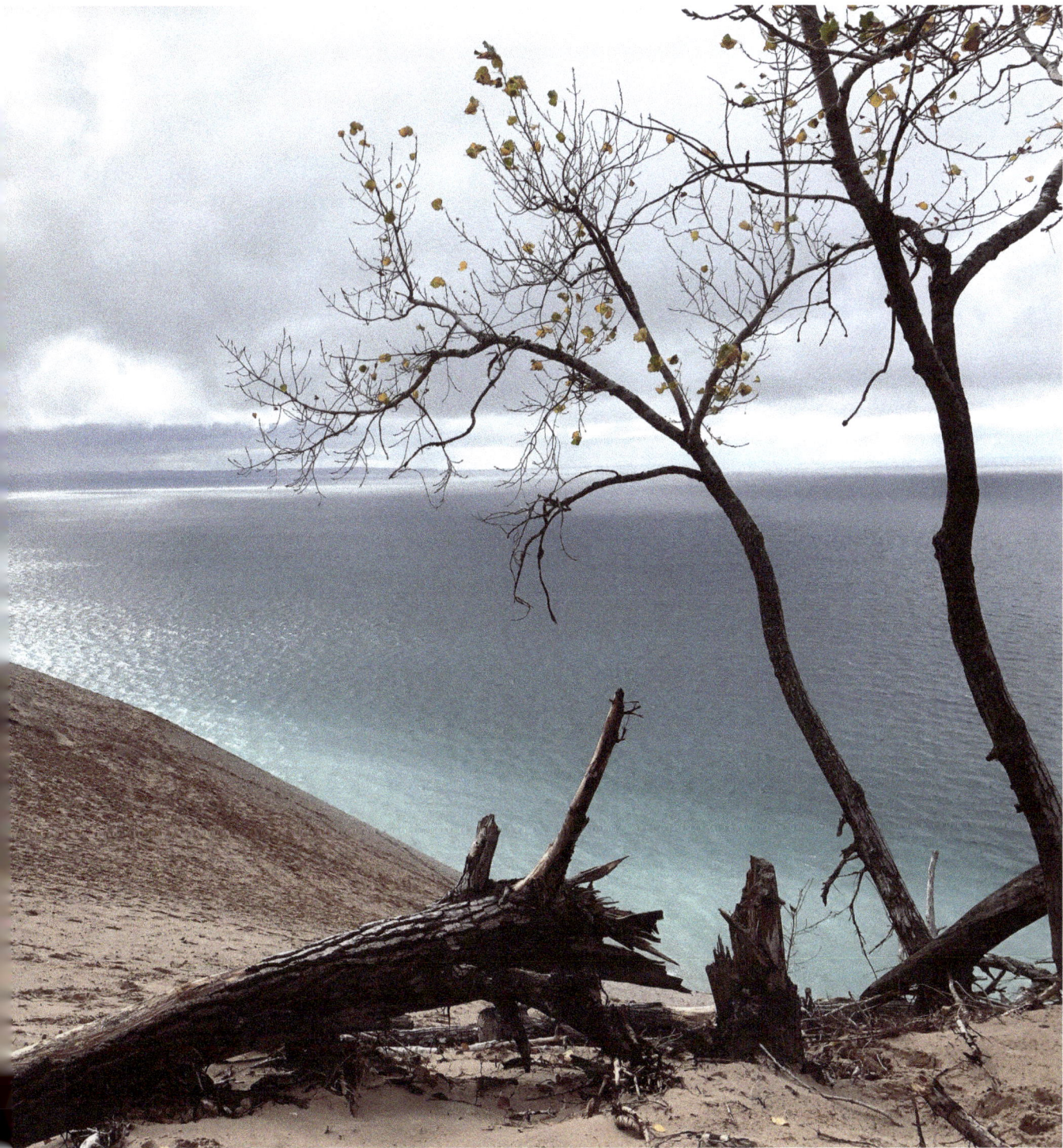

KAYAK RENTALS:

We have not had to use rented kayaks, but if you are visiting the area, here are some local rental shops:

- Crystal River Outfitters, Glen Arbor. (231) 334-4556. Rent kayaks for use on the Crystal River. They will deliver to your inland lake or river location.

- All About Water, Glen Arbor. (269) 214-4848. This company provides guided tours within the Sleeping Bear National Lakeshore and delivers kayaks and paddleboards to your Leelanau County location.

- North Shore Outfitters, Northport. (231)386-1222.

- Sleeping Bear Surf and Kayak, Empire. (231) 326-9283. Reservations on kayaks must be made the day prior as limited kayaks are available.

- Suttons Bay Bikes, Suttons Bay. (231) 421-6815. Kayaks and paddleboards with free delivery to all Leelanau County and West Traverse City areas.

- The River Outfitters, Traverse City. (231) 883-1413.

- Paddle TC, Traverse City. (231) 492-0223. If you are looking for a paddle along the West Grand Traverse south shoreline, this rental shop may be for you. They are located right at the Open Space, near the intersection of the Grandview Pkwy (US-31) and Union Street.

Michigan's official state motto is, *Si Quaeris Peninsulam Amoenam Circumspice,* which translates from the Latin to, "If you seek a pleasant peninsula, look about you". While I think the word "pleasant" is a bit of an understatement, if you are looking for a pleasant peninsula, you don't have to look any further than the Leelanau Peninsula. The little finger of the Michigan is a great place to explore in a kayak. Here is what we saw on our kayak trips around and in the Leelanau Peninsula and some tips on how you can do what we did.

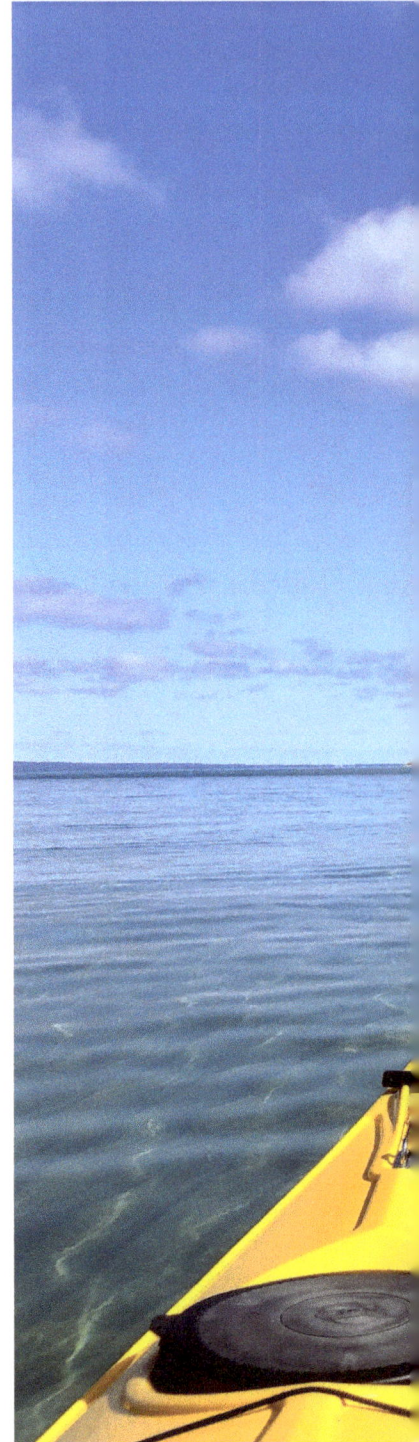

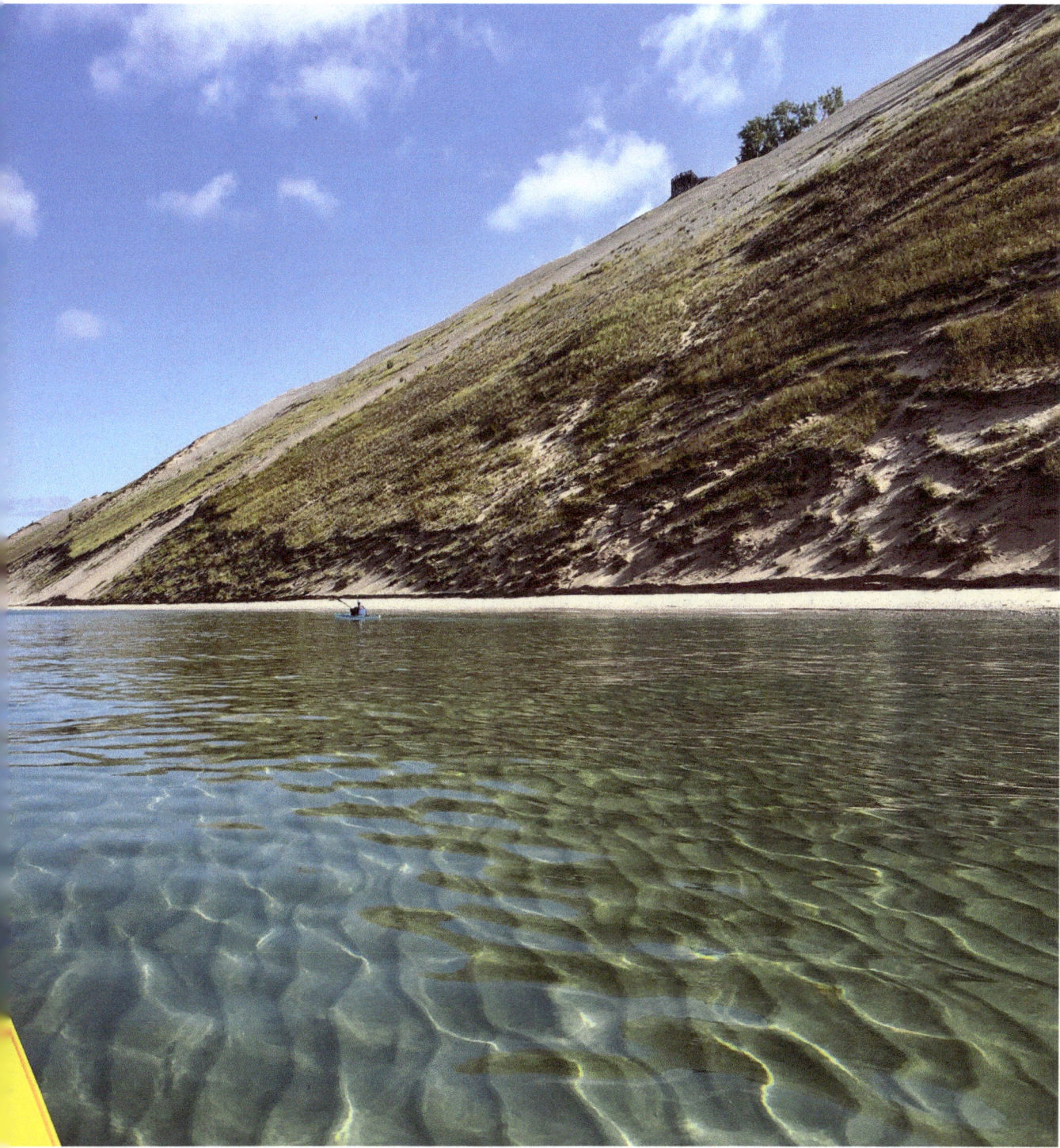

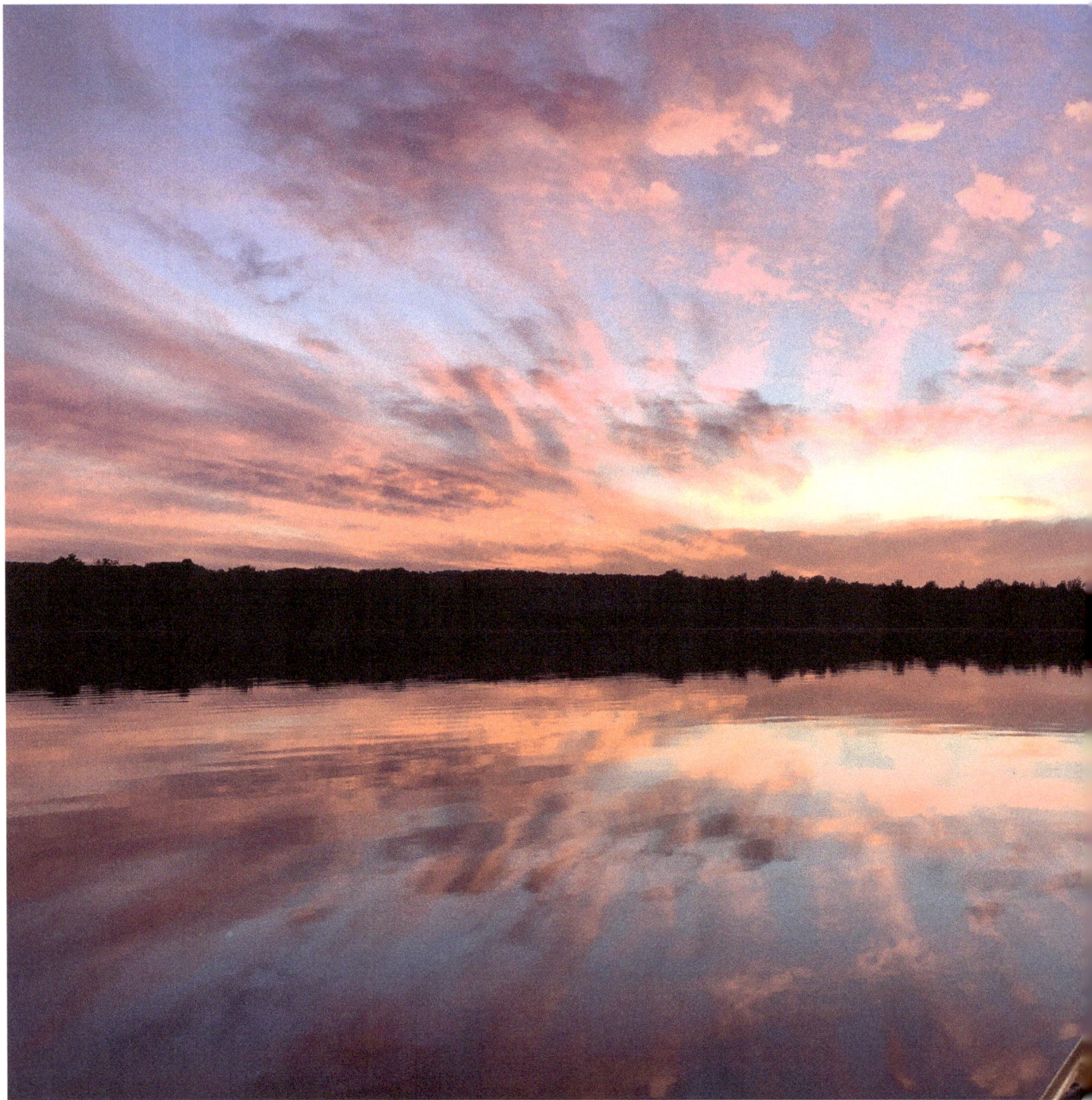

LAST WORDS

My personal history has roots in Leelanau that go way back to the mid-1960s, when my family vacationed several summers on Little Glen Lake. We visited the sand dunes that soon were to become the Sleeping Bear Dunes National Lakeshore. Later, after attending Hope College, I became a teacher in the Traverse City Area Public Schools. I eventually bought a home on Cedar Lake, in the southeast corner of Leelanau County. (I never knew the lake was even there, but I saw a house for sale on it on my way to a football coaching staff meeting at head coach Jim Ooley's house on nearby Regal Street. Well, I bought that house, met my future wife, Mary, and helped raise two wonderful daughters, Jody and Kacie, on Cedar Lake.) I enjoyed a 38-year career teaching social studies and coaching football and basketball at Traverse City Central High School. In retirement, one of the activities that I actively pursued was kayaking. At first, I only paddled in an inexpensive kayak on the lake just out my back door. Eventually I tried bigger and more distant waters.

I was the boys varsity basketball coach at Traverse City Central for 22 years, and my first junior varsity coach and varsity assistant coach was Larry Burns. On long bus rides to games, he often talked about his kayaking trips, like paddling with the killer whales out in Puget Sound. It sounded like a thrilling adventure to me. Eventually, after we had both retired from the Traverse City school system, we started kayaking more and more on the inland lakes around the Grand Traverse region. As our skills and equipment improved, we began venturing out on bigger inland lakes, and eventually out on Lake Michigan.

On each the trips, I would bring my iPhone and take pictures of whatever impressed me. I jokingly told Larry that he and I were the modern day kayaking duo of Butch Cassidy and the Sundance Kid. If you don't know the movie, Butch was the guy with the big plans, while Sundance was the better shooter. Larry's skills were better than mine (as Sundance's shooting skills were better than

Butch's), and Larry is also the one featured in most of the photos. I tell him that's because of his (Paul Newman) good looks — but the main reason is probably that he still has a flip phone, and I don't know if it even has an operating camera. After each trip, I would usually post a few pictures on Facebook for my friends to see. Often, I would get comments about how nice the pictures were, and how I should consider writing a book.

I always thought that if I ever wrote a book it would be about my experiences as a high school basketball coach. In 30 years of coaching (and 38 years of teaching), you get to see and experience a lot of things. There were many great players, great games, great seasons and just a lot of interesting stories. But that book never got written. As I reflect on this book I have written, I think that although there are many contrasts between coaching in a noisy gym and paddling on a quiet lake, there are some interesting similarities and parallels. Here are a few that come to mind:

» I really enjoy both basketball and kayaking. There is a saying: "Do what you love and love what you do." Feeling passionate about something and doing it is what life is all about.

» In coaching, it is important to have an understanding and supportive spouse or significant other. The nice thing about kayaking is that it is an activity that both of you can do together. My wife, Mary, and I often go kayaking together, and she has also been supportive when I go without her. Larry's wife, Shirley, has also been very supportive of our many kayaking trips. (Or could it be that they are both just happy to have us out of the house for a few hours?)

» Both coaching basketball and kayaking involve preparation, if you are going to do it correctly. In basketball, I had both a season plan and individual game plans. In kayaking, I plan out places prior to the kayaking season that would be fun to paddle. Individual day trips also get a "game plan".

» In basketball, even if you have prepared a good game plan, things happen that require that your plans be altered or dropped entirely. Halftime adjustments are important. In kayaking, conditions are also subject to change, and sometimes the plans for that day need to be adjusted too.

» Both coaching basketball and kayaking require the proper equipment. The team needs to be properly outfitted, and there is always new equipment being developed to improve the game. Kayaking is similar. If you don't know which kayak or piece of equipment is best for you, do some research or ask those kayakers with more experience what you need to have a safe and fun season.

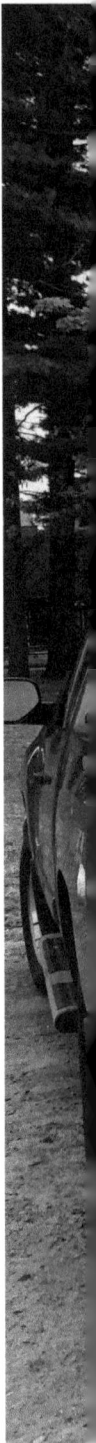

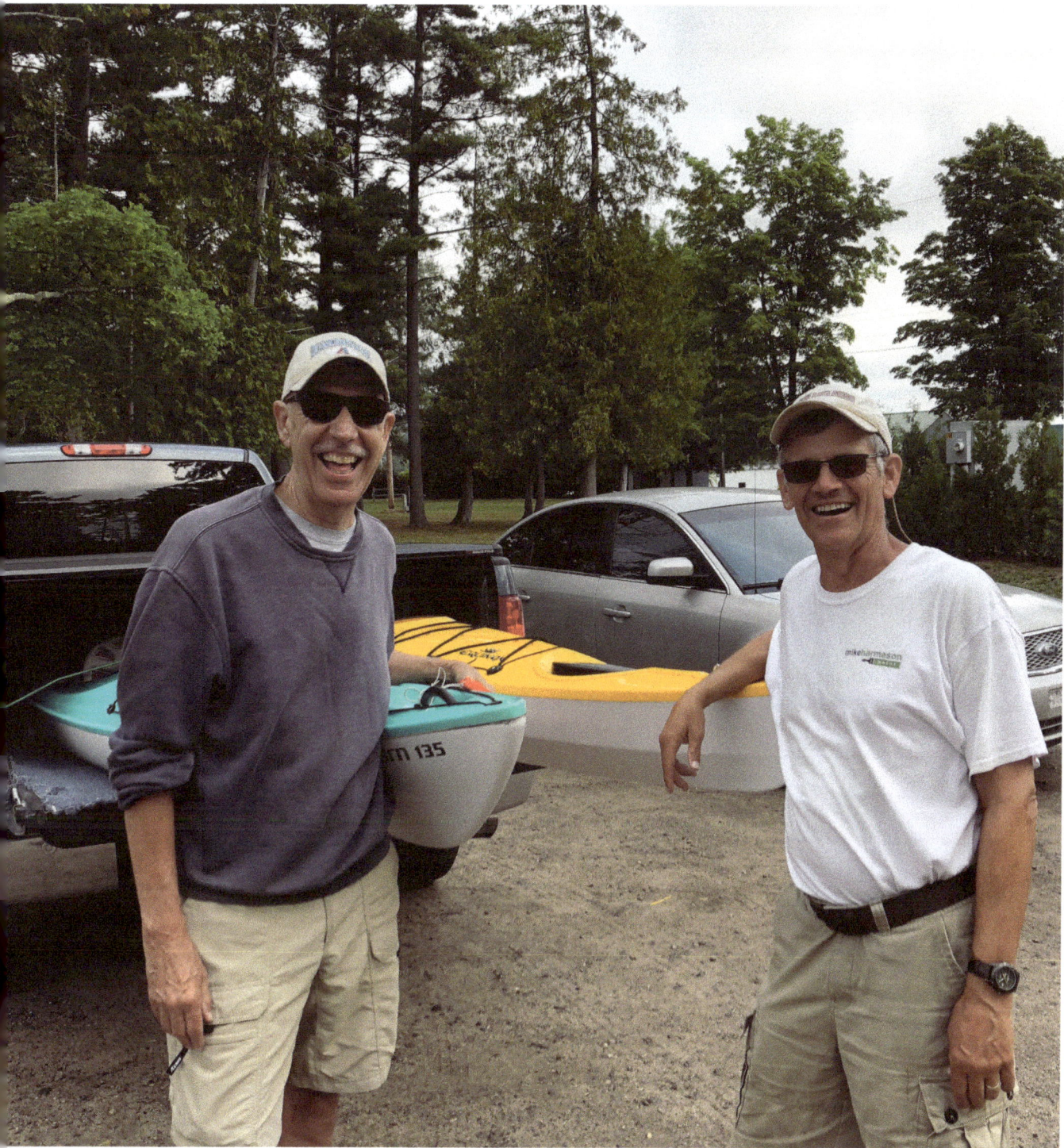

» Remember to enjoy the moment. In basketball, that meant keeping a perspective when things got rough. It was good to remember to enjoy each game and each season. There were bad calls, a few difficult parents and tough losses, but these aren't what I remember most. What I do remember are the relationships with players, coaches and other people involved in the game. I remember the thrills — both the great victories and the tough losses. In kayaking, problems can come up, and there can sometimes be difficult conditions to deal with, but it is important to be in the moment and enjoy each paddle.

» Each basketball season was like a separate journey. When the season ended, there was time to reflect on the year and enjoy an awards banquet to celebrate that journey — no matter the number of wins and losses. After each kayaking season, I always put together two photo books of our trips from that season from Shutterfly or Sam's Club Photo. At the end of each season, before Larry and Shirley leave for Arizona for the winter, we meet at one of our favorite pubs in Traverse City and have our "End of Season Banquet." I usually have the books back by then, and it is always great to relive each trip of that year.

» In keeping with the tradition of giving awards, here are my Leelanau Peninsula Day Trip Kayaking Award Winners. (Picking "winners" is very difficult. At the end of many a paddle, either Larry or I would comment that we had just paddled in a spectacular location — but where would it rank in the top 5 of the places in Leelanau?).

Here are some of my awards:

» Favorite Month to Paddle in Leelanau: September. Many of our best day trips—especially on Lake Michigan—have been in the month of September. The humidity tends to be lower, the temperatures are usually still nice and warm, there usually are many days with light winds (often in a row), and there are fewer people than in the busier months of summer.

» Favorite River: The upper reaches of the Crystal River.

» Favorite Medium-sized Inland Lake: Cedar Lake. The colors of the water and the fact it is so close to Traverse City still amaze me.

» Favorite Medium-sized Inland Lake Not Named Cedar Lake: Little Traverse Lake. I love the variety of things to see on this lake. The fact that Sugarloaf Mountain is in the background is an added bonus.

» Favorite Small Inland Lake: Shell Lake. Such a pretty, pristine lake. Off the beaten path, but It is worth the effort to paddle this little gem.

» Favorite Big Inland Lake: North Lake Leelanau. I just love the deep, blue-green colors of this big lake.

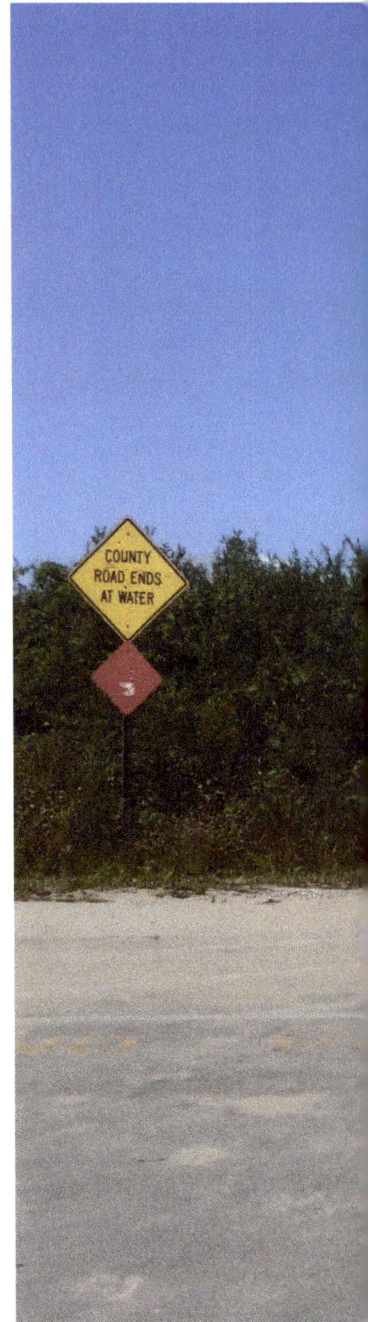

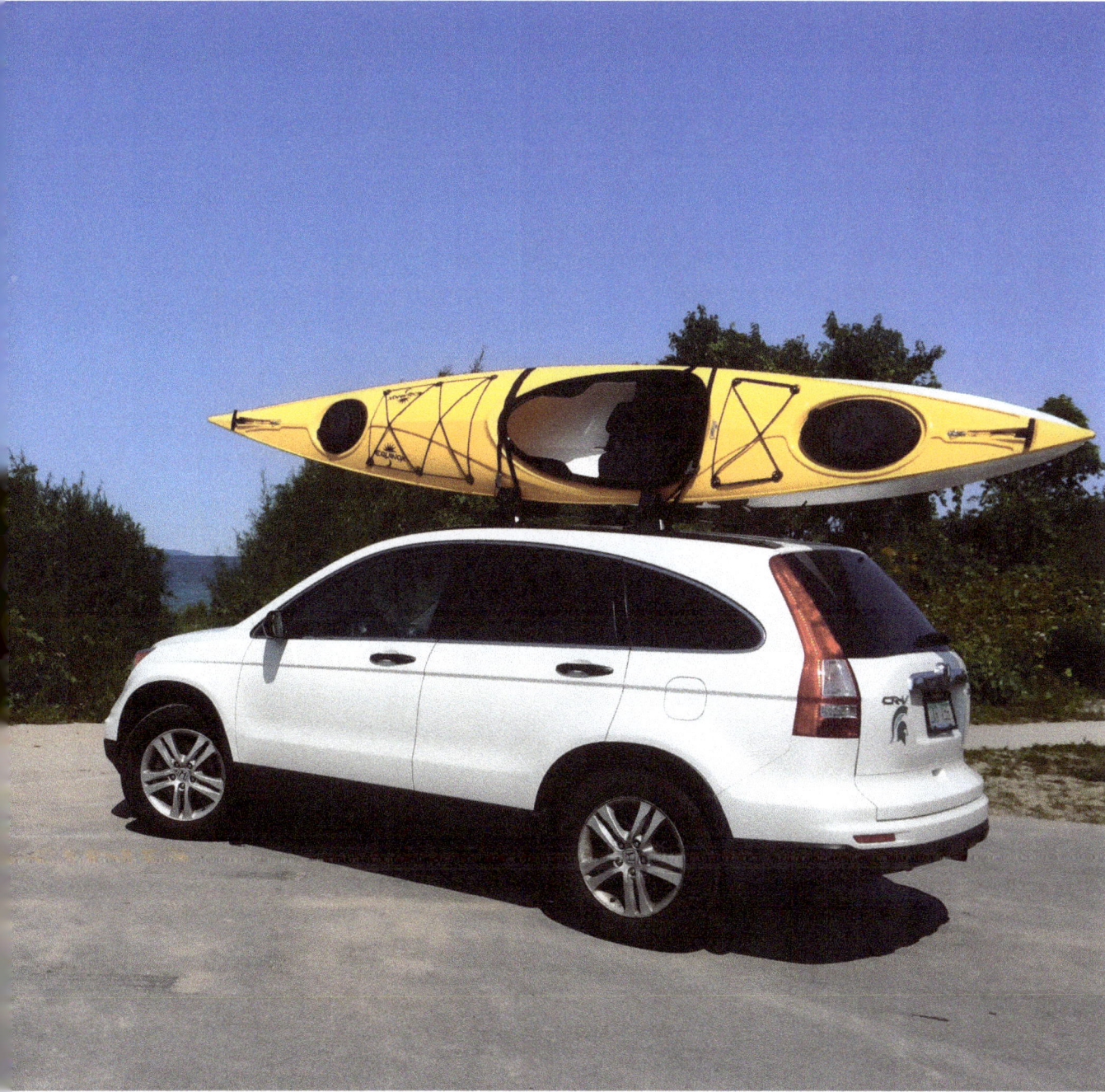

- » Favorite Sleeping Bear Dunes Shore: Sleeping Bear Dunes, Glen Haven to Empire. The views of the massive sand dunes on one side, the Manitous to the north and the expanse of Lake Michigan is just stunning.

- » Favorite Sleeping Bear Dunes Shore Runner-Up: Pyramid Point. This location never disappoints. The sun's shadows on the sand are so dramatic.

- » Favorite Lake Michigan Location (not in the Sleeping Bear Dunes): Gill's Pier to Cathead Point. I did not expect the real beauty of the water, submerged rocks and the pretty, but smaller dunes.

- » Favorite Lake Michigan Location (not in the Sleeping Bear Dunes) Runner-Up: Leland to the Clay Cliffs. The water just north of Leland is simply amazing. The actual Clay Cliffs were also dramatic and breathtaking.

- » Favorite Grand Traverse Bay Paddle: Northport to the Leelanau Lighthouse. You can almost feel the presence of those wooden steamers that would seek the protected harbor to get out of the storms. The view to the horizon, looking north and east, is an added bonus.

- » Favorite West Bay Location Runner-Up: Omena Bay. The colors of the deepest parts of the bay are almost purple. The historical significance of this area as an early mission, and those Civil War generals, also make it special for me as a history buff.

- » MVP (Most Valuable Paddle): Sleeping Bear Point to the Pierce Stocking Lookout. If I could only have one more paddle in my life, this would be where I would go.

- » Best Single Day: September 26, 2014. This paddle from Glen Haven to the Sleeping Bear capped an amazing week of unseasonably warm temperatures, no winds and cloudless skies. There were three trips to the National Lakeshore that week — The Platte River on the 23rd, Pyramid Point on the 24th, and finally the Big Bear on the 26th. These were the perfect conditions that kayakers dream about. I've never seen such a great stretch of weather.

- » Best Assists: Mary Constant and Shirley Burns. Thanks for letting us go on our "expeditions."

- » MVP (Most Valuable Paddler Award): Larry Burns. I would never have seen what I saw without Larry. Larry's experience and confidence gave me what I needed. Added bonus: we solved many of the world's problems on our paddles.

- » Luckiest and Most Thankful Paddler: Me. I love having a mental map of the wonderful waters of the Leelanau Peninsula. It is great to drive by areas, or look at a map of Leelanau and think, "Yes, we paddled here."

The Etymology of the word "Leelanau" has been debated by historians. One traditional explanation is that it was a Native American word for "delight of life." Another, currently more accepted, reason is that it was made up in the 1820s by Henry Schoolcraft, who was the US government's Indian Agent in Michigan. He made up many "Indian-sounding names" for many of Michigan's counties, like Alcona, Algoma, Allegan, Alpena, Arenac, Iosco, Kalkaska, Oscoda, and Tuscola. More recently, however, scholars are inclined to give credit to his Ojibwa and Scots-Irish wife, Jane Johnston Schoolcraft. She began using the name "Leelinau" as her pen name for her writings. I will leave the etymology issues and the actual source for "Leelanau" to others. For me, the first one just seems best for this book. Leelanau is definitely one of the "delights of life" for me — especially when I am out on her waters in my kayak.

I hope you have enjoyed our tour of Leelanau through this book and its pictures. If you are moved enough to try some of the day trips for yourself, maybe I will see you out there. May you have a delightful time and may your winds and conditions be favorable. Happy paddling!

Leelanau County has the second highest proportion of water to land of any county in the United States—coming in second only behind Keweenau County, Michigan. Not counting the places we have paddled more than once, our Leelanau kayak day trips has totaled 194.5 miles! This included 100 miles of Great Lakes shoreline; 8.9 miles of its rivers; and 85.6 miles around 16 of its inland lakes

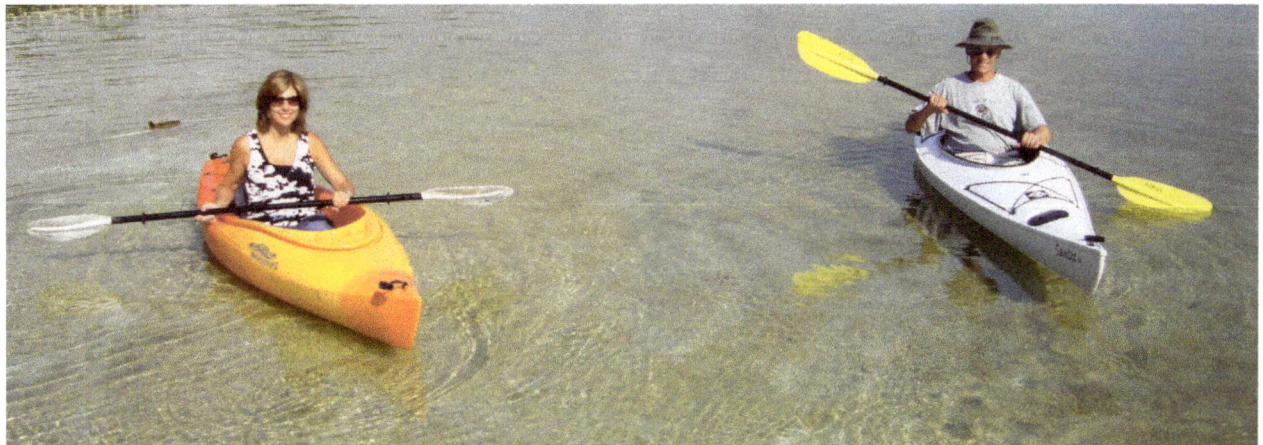

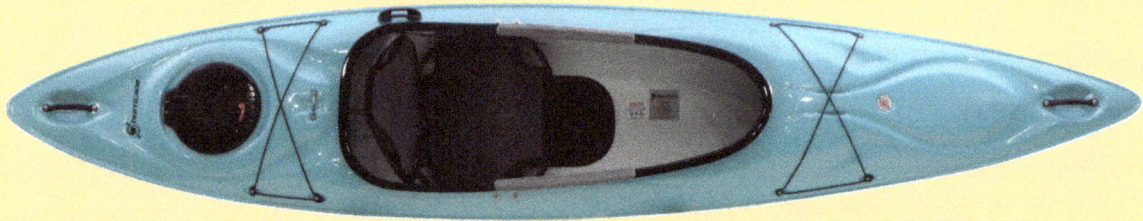

Go Wild

Santee 120 Sport
36 LBS. *
12'
*With the seat removed

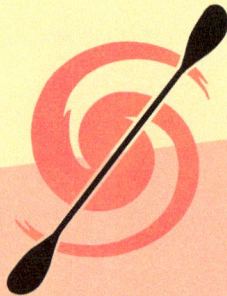

hurricane
Leaders in Lightweight
www.hurricaneaquasports.com

Sojourn 135
45 LBS.
13' 5"

Travel Light

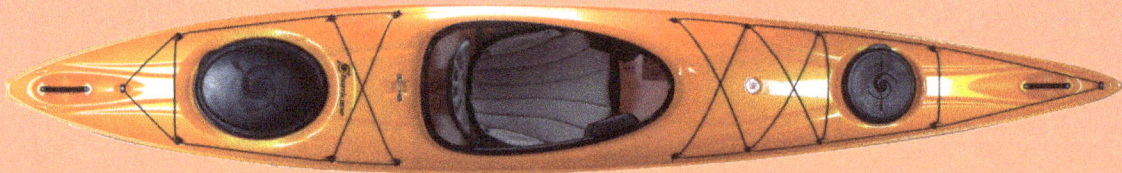

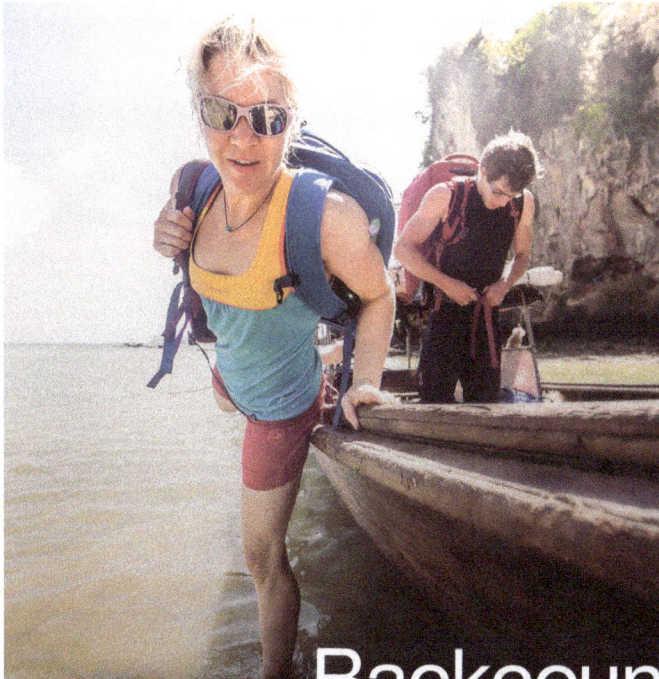

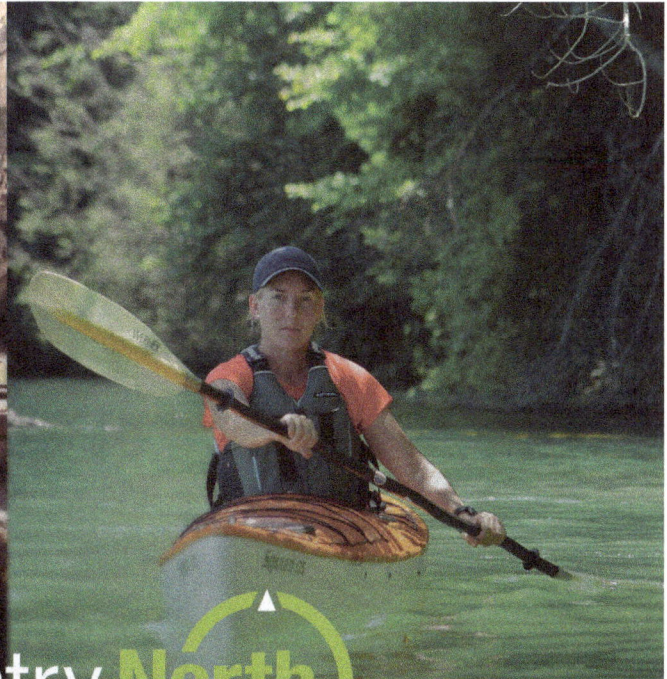

Backcountry North

TRAVEL. PADDLE. CAMP. EXPLORE.

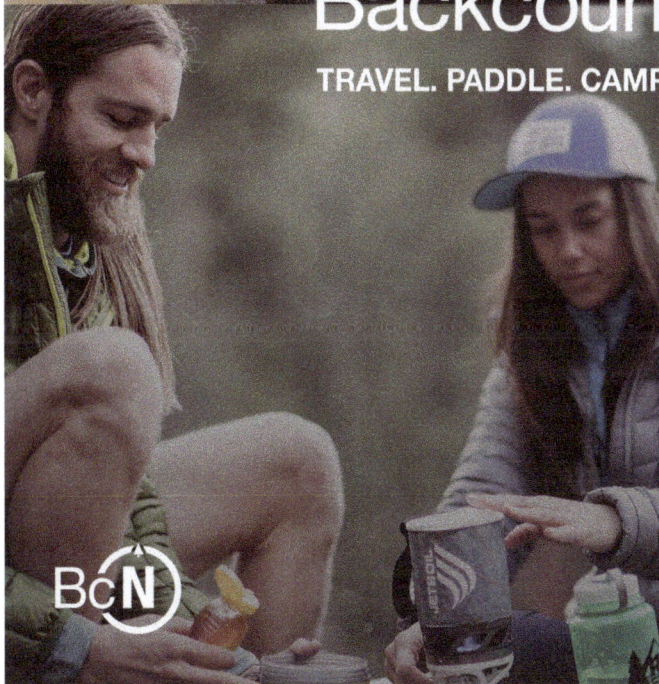

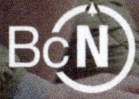

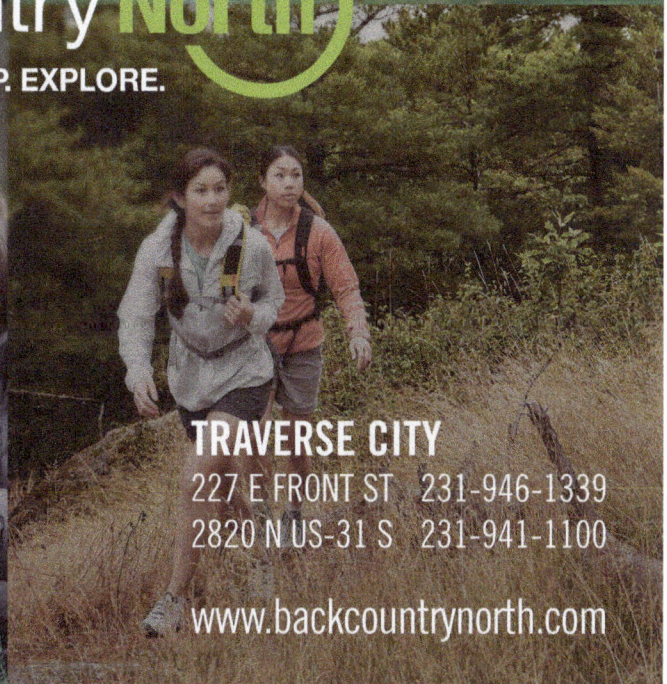

BcN

TRAVERSE CITY
227 E FRONT ST   231-946-1339
2820 N US-31 S   231-941-1100

www.backcountrynorth.com

www.ingramcontent.com/pod-product-compliance
Lightning Source LLC
Chambersburg PA
CBHW051319020426
42333CB00031B/3408

* 9 7 8 1 9 4 3 9 9 5 6 2 2 *